The Overfed Head

What others are saying about *The Overfed Head:*

I feel honored to review this great book. As someone who has brought "thintuition" into my life after dieting on and off for the last fifteen years, I have a great perspective. The honesty and candor of Rob Stevens in this book is refreshing. The thintuition approach will bring back the power and freedom in your life that has been lost around being overweight.

His concepts of getting in touch with or reconnecting to our bodies, honoring our needs, and being good to ourselves are so much more empowering than the limitations and restrictions set up by diets. It does require a change in thinking and a willingness to let go of some previous beliefs . . . but why not? If you're reading this, you, too, have probably been dieting for a while, and have not been as successful as you would have liked—or not successful at all.

I love thintuition, not only because I have lost twenty-five pounds and kept it off, but because I have lost my cynicism and resignation about weight loss as well. I have also lost more weight more easily than I ever thought possible. I love the freedom and confidence I have in my relationship to eating and in knowing my body. The power in that is amazing—the power that's missing in diet after diet.

As an obstetrician/gynecologist, I deal with the concerns about weight from a medical, as well as from an emotional and psychological standpoint. I have already recommended thintuition to many of my patients. Having women become empowered in their access to weight loss will lead to their success.

Leslie A. McCloskey, M.D.
Obstetrician/Gynecologist
Northwestern Memorial Hospital

Over the weekend, I read a stimulating and insightful book, titled *The Overfed Head* by Rob Stevens. The book describes Mr. Stevens' battle with morbid obesity, as he gained a variety of insights into his condition and, especially, began to realize the present lack of solutions to successful weight maintenance. Through what we'll call a "controlled clinical trial of one," Mr. Stevens listened to the "wee small voice within," stimulated substantially by prior insights gained from a seminal book by Robert Schwartz titled, *Diets Don't Work*. Mr. Stevens subsequently came up with the concept and, I believe, the reality of "thintuition."

The book documents the evolution of the process of thintuition through the perspectives gained from one or another of the author's unsuccessful attempts at weight loss. The fact is that much of what we all have been taught about weight loss actually results in *increased* weight. Over millions of years, the body has been evolving ways to store, retain, and then *not* lose weight and energy stores (fat). I fully agree with Mr. Stevens that diets are unsatisfactory, and often unhealthy, solutions to weight control!

The central concepts of thintuition are right on target! "Naturally thin" people, as Mr. Stevens characterizes them, and there are still some around (though increasingly few as the food industry wreaks its havoc with our thintuition), **simply eat when hungry, eat what they want and, most importantly, stop eating when they're not hungry.** These concepts are simple, straightforward, and accurate!

In the end, this book is well-written and fun to read! The examples given and the easy flow of the words and phrases make it a quick read and enhance one's ability to conceptualize the central themes of thintuition. I recommend that you simply sit down and read it, whether you're overweight or not!

John N. Sheagren, M.D.
Chair, Department of Internal Medicine
Advocate Illinois Masonic Medical Center,
and Professor of Medicine
University of Illinois, College of Medicine

♦ ♦ ♦

When I read *The Overfed Head*, I saw reflected in it many of the challenges my patients routinely face in my internal medicine practice, in which I specialize in weight management. Many of my patients fit the model of successfully losing weight, repeatedly on different diets, only to regain the weight lost once they go off those diets.

I have always struggled with how to best help my patients develop a healthy relationship with food and eating. I am always encouraging my patients to commit to a lifestyle change rather than to a temporary diet.

I routinely recommend many of the ideas Rob Stevens presents in *The Overfed Head*. Readers will find useful tools through which they can identify the reasons why they eat that have nothing to do with hunger. Readers will also discover a new way of thinking about food as fuel for their bodies, not as something to satisfy emotional needs, and to approach eating as a ceremonious and joyful occasion.

Coming from the perspective of one who has finally overcome his struggles with weight, Rob Stevens gives hope to those who are looking for a permanent solution. I believe that with true commitment, anyone can find success through his approach.

Laura L. Concannon, M.D.
Section Head, Department of Integrative Medicine
Advocate Illinois Masonic Medical Center,
and Assistant Professor of Medicine
University of Illinois, College of Medicine

I started reading *The Overfed Head* and couldn't put it down until I'd finished. What a compelling, logical, straightforward, enjoyable read! This book lays out an easy-to-follow, easy-to-implement way of thinking about eating that leads to effective weight loss. And I know it works, because it's worked for me. Great job, Rob Stevens!

Jeffrey A. Miller, M.S.W.
Psychotherapist and
Author, *The Anxious Organization*

The Overfed Head

What if everything you know about weight loss is wrong?

by Rob Stevens
Founder of thintuition

First Edition

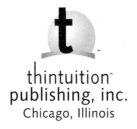

thintuition™
publishing, inc.
Chicago, Illinois

Published by:
thintuition™ publishing, inc.
P.O. Box 180182
Chicago, IL 60618
www.thintuition.com

ISBN   0-9746542-0-5
Library of Congress Control Number (LCCN): 2004103918
First Printing 2004
Printed and bound in the United States of America
Cover design and illustrations by Dirk I. Tiede and Andy Crestodina

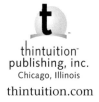

thintuition
publishing, inc.
Chicago, Illinois
thintuition.com

Notice

The information contained in this book is general in scope and is intended only to assist people in their personal weight loss and weight management efforts. The information provided in this book is not to be considered medical advice and should not be interpreted as a substitute for a medical consultation, evaluation, diagnosis or treatment by a physician. All information contained in this book should be viewed only as the opinion and belief of the author.

Before beginning this or any weight loss or weight management program, or before undertaking any of the recommendations provided in this book, you are urged to seek the advice of a physician or health practitioner. Never disregard professional medical advice or delay in seeking it because of something you have read in this or any book. Individuals with *any* health concerns are specifically warned to seek professional medical advice prior to initiating any form of weight loss or weight management program.

The author, publisher, and distributor disclaim any liability or loss, personal or otherwise, resulting from anyone following any of the recommendations in this book.

Contents

Chapter 1
Results Not Typical

This is probably not the first weight loss book you've read that begins with a before-and-after story. From the back cover photo you will have already gathered that at one time I was obese, and that now I'm not. You will have surmised that I'm going to tell you how I lost the weight and how you, too, can achieve the same happy result. If you are not skeptical at this point, you ought to be. My success is no guarantee at all of your success. My hope is that this book will disabuse you forever of the notion that having lost a lot of weight makes someone an expert on how *you* should lose weight. If you're presently heavier than you want to be, chances are such "experts" are a part of your problem.

Losing a lot of weight on a diet is not an unusual accomplishment. You've probably done it yourself—perhaps many times. What is unusual about me is that I *stopped* dieting in 1998, lost 140 pounds over the course of the following year and a half, and have kept it off ever since. You're probably assuming that instead of a diet, I made a permanent change in my eating habits. And you're right. I started eating what I actually wanted to eat. If you were to raid my refrigerator right now, you'd find real butter, real mayonnaise, real sugar—none of that reduced-fat, reduced-calorie gunk I used to inflict on myself when I was heavy.

Yes, I know that sounds unbelievable. For twenty-five years, I shared the belief that certain foods have the power to make you fat or thin. It was my *belief system* about food—*not* the foods themselves—that kept me overweight. When I changed my thinking, I was able to shed the weight and keep it off, without a struggle.

The wealth of data we possess on diet, nutrition, and weight control is astounding. More of it has been produced in our lifetimes than was produced in the entire previous history of human civilization. Walk into any bookstore and you'll find a whole wall of the stuff. You can't channel surf for ten minutes or glance at a newspaper without encountering some new info on what you should and shouldn't be eating. Legions of people now make their living as diet counselors, nutritionists, and trainers—professions that scarcely existed a generation ago. We also have a host of new food products meant to keep us slim: low-fat, non-fat and artificially sweet. And yet we're in the midst of an obesity epidemic. A majority of Americans are overweight, and a great many of them are dangerously so.

You might suppose that the problem of overweight is driving the growth of the diet industry, that it has sprung up to serve an obvious need. But what if the *opposite* is actually the case? What if all this data, all these products and services, are actually contributing to the problem? It's clear that the more we've learned about fat, the fatter we've gotten. Might that be because everything we think we've learned is actually wrong? That is the hypothesis I'd like you to consider.

You won't find any testimonials in this book. Although I know many others who have succeeded with the approach I'll be describing, I won't be telling you their before-and-after stories. The experiences of other people are really beside the point. The essence of the approach I call "thintuition" is learning to tune in to your own experience. If you come to agree that what I'm saying makes sense, you will perhaps act on the idea and discover for yourself whether it works for you. Your own success story is the only one that matters. I begin with my story mainly to describe the faulty assumptions that guided all my previous attempts to lose weight, and the repetitive failures that resulted.

I was about ten years old when I went on my first diet. Although I wasn't yet seriously overweight, both my older sister and father already had weight problems. My parents must have figured that my childhood pudginess was a sign of bigger trouble to come. Like so many well-meaning parents of chubby kids, they set me on a course that pretty much guaranteed a lifelong struggle with fat. I don't fault them for this. They didn't know any better. Back then, nobody did.

My father was a holocaust survivor who had experienced real anxiety about where the next meal was coming from. This childhood experience of scarcity left a deep impression that subsequent abundance could never entirely erase. Safe in the Land of Plenty, my father continued to regard food as a limited resource that must not be wasted. The unspoken but clearly understood rule at our house was to finish everything on our plates. My sister and I learned by example that leaving food was simply not an option. Being full was no excuse for throwing away good food. Curiously, my parents never made the connection between my clean plate and my thickening waistline. Instead, my mother stocked up on low-calorie foods, and I went on dutifully consuming every last bite of cottage cheese and carrots.

The food served officially at the family dinner table was more than enough to satisfy my physical hunger, but not my appetite for treats, so I supplemented (and subverted) the healthy diet my mother had put me on out of my own pocket money. Now it was "fun" food that was scarce, and I was still very much my father's son. Fast food bargains attracted me irresistibly. Four burgers for a dollar? That was an opportunity not to be missed. With a familiar sense of duty, I'd wolf down all four, hungry or not.

Although I overate throughout my teens, I continued to think of myself as "husky" or "chunky" rather than fat. Luckily, I wasn't heavy enough during my high school years to be socially isolated by my weight. I was a pretty popular kid, and nobody picked on me. But by the end of my first year of college, I was undeniably fat, and unhappy about it. That year, I experienced my first romantic rejection. In the depression that followed, I turned to food for comfort. I found myself in that conundrum so familiar to the overweight: feeling that fat was the source of my unhappiness and that food was the remedy.

From then on, dieting became a way of life for me. It ruled my life and consumed my thoughts. Since my first diet at the age of ten, I estimate that I went on an average of eight diets a year and spent a cumulative total of thirteen years on some diet or other. And the irony of it is, I'd have to say I was a *successful* dieter: successful in the sense that I often met my goal weight. Over the years, I lost, regained and lost again *hundreds* of pounds. Because I managed to reach my goal on

some diets—often losing sixty to seventy pounds at a time—
I continued to believe that, given the right circumstances,
dieting worked. Unconsciously, I believed (as many people
do) that all I had to do was to find the *right* diet: the miracle
diet to end all diets.

In search of that miracle, I embraced every new diet idea
that came along. From counting calories, I shifted to counting
fat grams and then to counting carbs. I could give you the full
nutritional rundown on every food item in the supermarket.
The Atkins Diet—like any approach that "allows" you to eat
unlimited quantities of a certain food group—had great
appeal for me. What's not to love about guilt-free bacon? At
some level, I believed that it probably wasn't healthy to shun
one food group while overindulging in another, but I wanted
to be thin more than I wanted to be healthy. It was short-term
discomfort—dehydration, lightheadedness, and a perpetual
case of constipation—rather than concern for the long-term
consequences that caused me to abandon the Atkins
approach.

Between serious commitments to diets named after doctors,
I had many fad diet flings. The most short-lived was one of
those miracle combination diets where you have to follow an
exact menu on day one, then a different menu on day two,
and so forth. On day three, I had to eat beets. No substitutions

were possible. The diet specifically indicated that beets eaten on day three would cure my sluggish metabolism. I loathe beets. The Cabbage Soup diet was another desperate measure I wasn't quite desperate enough to adopt for long. Still, I have no doubt that, had I persisted with beets or cabbage soup, I'd have lost weight. Even really stupid diets will prevent you from overeating if you stick with them consistently.

Over the years, I came to acknowledge that there were certain things I was never going to do consistently. You can put up with just about anything if you know it's temporary, but I could not resign myself to the idea of giving up foods I love and filling up with foods I dislike *for life.* The reward for every dieting success was being able to go off the diet. Again and again I reached my goal weight—and maintained it for about a day. I celebrated every diet success with festive overindulgence in all the favorite foods I'd had to give up. Not surprisingly, I soon gained back all the weight—and then some.

The program that worked best for me was Weight Watchers. Its balance appealed to my common sense, and its flexibility worked well with my lifestyle. I managed to stick with it for eight months and lost seventy pounds. Having achieved my goal weight (185 pounds back then) by a method I found relatively painless (relative to eating beets or being constipated, at any rate), I felt like a Weight Watchers success story. However, I went off the regime and within a few weeks was already regaining the weight. A year later, I weighed 270 pounds—fifteen pounds more than I'd weighed when I began the program.

In the discouragement that followed every diet, I sometimes toyed with giving up dieting for good. The "fat acceptance" movement had some persuasive points to make and accorded well with my natural tendency to look on the bright side. The fact was that other people already did accept me, fat or thin. When overweight, I fell comfortably into the role of "the funny fat guy." Yet deep down I felt that to accept my obesity was to settle for being less than my best self. I knew that being fat was holding me back in many aspects of my life. Never mind what other people thought—when I looked in the mirror, *I* didn't like what I saw. Despite having been overweight most of my life, this fat self didn't look or feel to me like my real self, my natural self.

And that presented me with a dilemma, because the relatively thin person I was at the end of each successful diet didn't seem natural or real either. My pared-down shape felt temporary somehow, overshadowed by my dread of getting fat again. Regardless of whether I was binging or dieting, I was obsessed with food. What I really wanted was to enjoy my life—*and* my food—without having to think about it constantly. Diets only work if you remain on a diet forever. Nowadays this staying-on-a-diet-forever is referred to as a "lifestyle change." Call it what you like: It is still a diet. Who can be happy about being perpetually on a diet? How can we think of that as natural?

Exasperated with dieting, I turned to exercise as a possible solution. Maybe if I got my metabolism going and burned a whole lot of calories, I'd be able to stay reasonably thin without having to deprive myself constantly. I joined a gym and signed up for a session with a personal trainer. After weighing me, he refused to let me work out until I'd obtained written permission from a physician. Not that I would have succeeded anyhow. Having to run for an hour to burn off the calories in one donut is not what I'd call an expedient solution. Exercising to get strong and vigorous is a great idea, and working out for this reason can be immensely pleasurable. Compulsively exercising to get or stay thin, though, is just a variation on compulsive dieting.

Diets only work if you remain on a diet forever.

The moment of truth

Many overweight people have what I call a "break-through moment" when they realize that they simply can't stand it any more, and they seriously resolve to change. For some it might be a health scare such as a coronary episode. For others it might be an embarrassing incident such as being asked to purchase two seats on a flight.

My own breakthrough came when I realized that despite my dramatic ups and downs, my overall trend had been to gain an average of ten pounds a year. By then, I was at my all time heaviest: over 300 pounds. Might have been as much as 315—I'm not sure, because past 300, I'd refused to get on a scale. I did the math and realized where all this was leading. Although I wasn't yet suffering any serious health consequences, I was by now well into the morbidly obese range. And at the rate of ten more pounds each year, I was on my way to being just plain gross. I didn't want to be that grotesquely fat guy. That wasn't me. I needed to change immediately, and forever. I wasn't willing to put up with another year of being obese, much less a lifetime of it.

At the same time, I realized that this annual ten-pound weight gain had been proceeding grimly, year in, year out, despite the fact that I spent an average of eight months out of every year on some diet or other. As I put it to myself then, I was getting fatter and fatter *despite* dieting. Now I recognize that I was getting fatter and fatter *because* of dieting, but that's getting a little ahead of my story. The point for me, in that breakthrough moment, was that dieting didn't work. If it hadn't worked for the first twenty-five years I'd done it, what would be different about the next twenty-five years? I decided to give it up for good.

On the face of it, this breakthrough didn't look entirely logical. On one hand, I was resolving firmly never to be fat again. On the other hand, I was resolving with equal firmness never to diet again. If I didn't diet, what was I going to do instead?

My solution at the time was to focus on eating healthfully. From my years of compulsive dieting, I already knew a great deal about the nutritional properties of food. I decided to apply this knowledge to a "permanent lifestyle change." I would eat balanced, healthy meals, and *only* balanced healthy meals, every day for the rest of my life. I would steer a sane middle course between the extremes of self-denial and self-indulgence that had, till then, governed my eating.

I figured my weight would gradually come to reflect this middle way. I would probably never be slim, but I could at least reverse my steady decline into morbid obesity.

I don't know how this would have worked over the long term. It was the best idea I'd ever come up with on my own, and I managed to stick with it for four or five months. Though I wasn't on what I called a "diet," I had succeeded in losing about forty pounds. Perhaps I truly would have kept my resolution for life, for it was certainly more keep-able than previous resolutions, and I was very determined. Yet my program still fell a bit short of my true desire—to enjoy my life *and* my food without having to fuss over it all the time. It is possible this desire would eventually have reasserted itself, leading back to my old cycle of careless eating, overindulgence, weight gain, and despair. I'll never know, for as fate would have it, my sane and reasonable idea was supplanted by a truly brilliant one. I discovered a way to attain my true desire: to have my cake, and a trim, healthy body besides.

While staying overnight at a friend's house, my mother had casually picked up a book about weight loss she found on the nightstand. She doesn't have a weight problem herself, but there was nothing else to read, and the title arrested her. It was *Diets Don't Work,* by Dr. Bob Schwartz. Knowing I'd recently come to the same conclusion, she figured it might interest me.

"Interest" is too mild a word. In mounting excitement, I devoured the copy she bought for me. Schwartz offered compelling evidence that diets don't work for anyone (i.e., not just me). He confirmed my own inkling that diets don't merely fail, but that in the long run they exacerbate the problem. I already knew that I was fat despite dieting, but by the end of his book, I finally understood that dieting had contributed to making me fatter. It was a whole lot worse than useless.

If Schwartz had merely strengthened my own resolve never to diet again, I'd have been grateful to have found his book. But he went on to offer an alternative solution much better than the one I was attempting to implement on my own. He noticed that medical studies on how to get thin almost always focused on the behavior of heavy people. It seemed to him that if you wanted to be thin, it would be better to study what thin people do.

So he started to observe people who had been slim all their lives. One thing he noticed immediately was that thin people seemed oblivious to the idea that some foods were fattening. Calories, fats, and carbohydrates never entered into their consideration when deciding what to eat. Indeed, many of them were quite clueless as to the nutritional content of foods. There was no particular pattern to what thin people, as a group, put into their bodies. Some ate traditionally balanced meals, while others lived on sweets or fast food. Some ate lots of meat while others ate lots of bread and pasta. The only common denominator was that, whatever they were eating, it wasn't making them fat. Exercise didn't seem to be a factor either. Some were very active, and some seemed to have a lot of nervous energy, but an equal number of thin people were slow-moving and sedentary. Some even managed to live confined to a wheelchair without putting on weight.

If not diet or exercise, what was it that all these naturally thin people had in common? Oddly enough, Schwartz found they were most like each other in their lack of reflection about what and why they ate. Ask heavy people why they ate what they did at their last meal, and you'll usually get a pretty longwinded answer. They'll tell you in depth and detail why it was good for them, or why, if it wasn't good for them, they ate it anyway. Ask a thin person and the almost universal response is to shrug and say, *"I was hungry."* Ask an overweight person at noon what they'd like for dinner, and they've usually got a good idea. Ask a thin person the same thing, and they don't seem to comprehend the question. A thin person may be keenly interested in food when they are hungry, but the moment their hunger is satisfied, the whole subject fades into oblivion for them. In short, the main difference Schwartz found between the naturally thin and the overweight was in how—and how much—they thought about food, eating, and weight.

As it happened, my roommate at that time was naturally thin. I found her at once enviable and perplexing. While my side of the fridge was stocked with fresh veggies, low-fat dressings, high fiber breads and the like, Dana's idea of a staple was full-fat chocolate fudge ice cream.

Where I carefully planned each nutritionally balanced meal and ate it at the regularly appointed time, Dana's eating seemed to follow no discernible pattern. At random intervals she would suddenly announce, "I'm hungry," then ask herself aloud, "Hmm, what sounds good right now?" If it was 7 p.m. and Cheerios appealed to her, Cheerios she would have. Once in a while she would declare herself hungry but have no answer to the follow-up question of what sounded good. On those occasions, she would decide to wait until she felt hungry enough to want something specific. Around eating, her only rule seemed to be to please herself, precisely and completely.

When, inspired by Schwartz's book, I began to observe Dana more closely, I discovered that she was *extremely* precise in the way she pleased herself. She would open that pint of chocolate fudge ice cream, take a spoonful and really

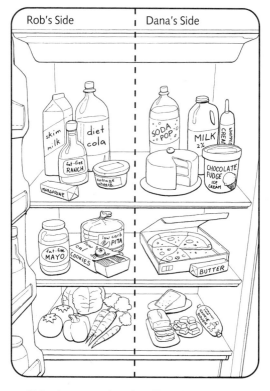

"Maybe one day they'll make carrots
that taste like fudge."

savor it, eyes closed, bliss spreading across her face. After a bite or two, she'd reseal the carton and return it reverently to the freezer. A pint would last her at least a week, and often longer. She'd open a bag of chips, eat a handful, and then forget about the rest till they'd gone stale. To throw away two-thirds of a bag of uneaten chips didn't seem to bother her at all. When I asked her why she left so much nice food unfinished, she never gave staying slim as her reason. She'd just say, "It hit the spot. I'm not hungry any more."

Schwartz's conclusion about what keeps naturally thin people thin was amazingly simple. It goes like this: Thin people eat only when hungry. Thin people eat exactly what they are hungry *for*. Thin people stop eating as soon as their hunger is satisfied. He went on to suggest that if overweight people were to adopt these three behaviors consistently, they would cease to be overweight.

So that's what I did. Compared with what I'd been doing previously, it was a cinch. I went on eating a lot of the healthy foods I'd been eating before, because I'd actually come to enjoy them. But I gave a pass to foods that had nothing going for them—to me, at least—except their nutritional virtue. No beets. No carrot sticks. No cabbage soup. For the first time in my adult life, I indulged *guiltlessly* in my favorites—pizza, nachos, and pastries. I discovered that a single slice of pizza, when fully savored, gave me more satisfaction than I used to get from polishing off the whole pie. Having assured myself that I could eat the foods I like best whenever I was hungry for them, I ceased to crave them. I had finally achieved my true desire—to simply enjoy eating, without having to obsess about it. For the first time in my life, I felt like I was fully in charge of my eating. I was free of the "shoulds" that had governed my choices while dieting and the rebellion against all these "shoulds" that had driven my sporadic binges. I felt like I was finally honoring my body's needs and treating myself with respect. My newfound self-esteem spread to other aspects of my life. I was handling *everything* more assertively and confidently, not just food.

On an emotional level this approach was so satisfying, that I probably would have persisted with it even if I wasn't losing much weight. But in fact, I was losing steadily. On my more optimistic diets, my goal weight had always been 185 pounds. That's still pretty hefty for a person of my height and build, but having been heavy all my life, I couldn't conceive of myself as any thinner. Once I passed the 300-pound mark, I'd have been happy to settle for anything under 200 pounds. This time I got down to 185 and kept losing. Wasn't trying to. It just happened. I finally stabilized at my true ideal weight of 160 and have remained there since 1999. I no longer own any of the larger-sized clothes I used to keep as back-up, for I no longer feel there's anything precarious about being thin. The size I am now is the size I fully expect to be for the rest of my life. I haven't the slightest desire to deviate from the behaviors that are keeping me thin, because these behaviors now come naturally to me and make me happy.

I had finally achieved my true desire—to simply enjoy eating, without having to obsess about it.

If this is such a great idea, why isn't everyone doing it?

Bob Schwartz's book was a bestseller, and the main idea expressed by its title, *Diets Don't Work,* entered the mainstream in a big way. Yet the American preoccupation with dieting has grown explosively since its publication. You will now routinely hear diet experts parroting the mantra "Diets don't work," then going on to spell out what, when, and how much you should eat. For "diet" they have merely substituted the euphemism "permanent lifestyle change." You are told to banish junk foods from your pantry forever, to resign yourself to low-fat, low-calorie, or low-carb substitutes for your favorite foods forever, to exercise daily forever, to stop eating three hours before bedtime forever, to monitor portion sizes forever, and so forth. This is the same old same old sensible advice that doesn't work because few people can follow it forever. The point is that if you are following rules about what, when, and how much to eat, you are on a diet, regardless of what you choose to call it.

In accepting the idea that diets don't work while continuing to go on diets that they no longer refer to as diets, most of the people who have been influenced by Schwartz seem to have missed the boat on the solution he was presenting. His greatest contribution, as I see it, was not his observation that diets don't work (which was really just a statement of the obvious) but the practical alternative he offered. Relatively few of his readers have been willing and/or able to adopt the behaviors of the naturally thin. Having gotten such great results myself, I began to wonder why more people weren't picking up his approach and running with it. After several years of reflecting on the matter, I believe I have identified the most common obstacles and what might be done to remove them.

Let me say at the outset that I have little to add to Schwartz's simple three-part formula. Eat only when you're hungry, eat exactly what you feel like eating, and stop eating when you stop being hungry. That is really and truly all it takes to achieve a weight that is healthy for you and maintain it for life. Both the beauty and the effectiveness of the idea lie in its simplicity, and for me to embellish on it would not be helpful. If you get it, believe it, and are, at this moment, able to actually do it, you can stop reading right now. The reason I am writing this book is that most overweight people have a lot of trouble either getting it, believing it, or doing it.

Getting it

So what's not to get? The idea is so simple, an infant could grasp it. In fact, infants do grasp it. Have you ever met a baby who didn't cry to be fed when hungry and lose all interest in suckling once satisfied? All of us are born knowing what we need, how much of it we need, and when we need it. Knowing this, and acting on it, is completely natural for both animals and human beings. We are all born with the instincts of the naturally thin—the instincts I call "thintuition." Some lucky people manage to retain this natural thintuition into adulthood and maintain a moderate, healthy weight all their lives. If you are overweight, you lost it at some point, and probably pretty early in your childhood. Losing touch with our natural instincts around food is an

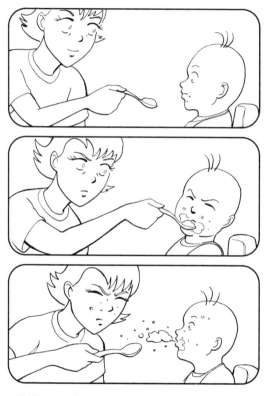

"Why can't he learn to clean his plate?"

almost universal aspect of our social conditioning.

Early on, most of us learn that meals are served at fixed intervals. By the time we are weaned, we've caught on to the idea that food is not always provided at the exact moment we want it, and that we are sometimes expected to eat it at moments when we don't want it. Learning to conform to this external schedule is the path of least resistance. We learn to disregard hunger that crops up at inopportune times and to eat when expected to eat, even if we don't feel hungry. Instead of being prompted to eat by the physical sensation of hunger, our eating becomes triggered by the clock and by the presence of food. If dessert is presented as the reward for cleaning our plates, we learn that foods considered good for us must be consumed to the point of satiety before we get to taste the foods we really desire. We learn to enjoy yummy foods despite feeling full because it's when we're already full that the yummies are usually served.

All of this learning has happened on an unconscious level by the time we reach school age. As we get older—and nowadays, not very much older—we also acquire a lot of conscious information about food. We learn that food is supposed to give you energy, that food makes you fat if you don't burn it all off, that you will get various disgusting diseases if you don't eat enough "good" food, and that you will get other terrible diseases if you eat too much "bad" food. Children in Africa have big bellies from not eating enough good food. Children in America have big bellies from eating too much bad food. If Brussels sprouts are a good food and French fries are a bad food, our instinctive preferences are probably not a reliable guide to avoiding a big belly. To know what's good and bad, you have to rely on what doctors, scientists, parents, and teachers tell you. You have to learn about things like vitamins, calories, proteins, and fats.

In short, we've spent our whole lives learning the precise opposite of eat when you're hungry, eat what you want, and stop eating when you're not hungry any more. What is perfectly obvious to every infant on the planet strikes us as utterly preposterous when we hear it as an adult.

We are all born with the instincts of the naturally thin—the instincts I call "thintuition."

Believing it

So naturally you have trouble believing it. Your head is already jam-packed with contrary information. Maybe what you've been reading for the past few minutes has sounded pretty convincing. But I can almost guarantee that before today is over, you'll turn on the television or open a magazine and be told that a certain kind of food makes you fat, or that you'll never lose weight if you're not exercising thirty minutes a day, or that your best hope is a gastric bypass operation. If Schwartz had been a voice crying in a wilderness, he might actually have been heard. But the voice of one author—even a bestselling author—is difficult to hear over the din of umpteen thousand diet experts.

Maybe you also have trouble believing because it just plain sounds too good to be true. How can the solution to a problem you've been studying and struggling with for years be so ridiculously simple? How can it be so seemingly painless? How can it possibly be true that you could lose weight by consistently pleasing yourself? After all, it was by pleasing yourself that you put on all those extra pounds in the first place, wasn't it?

No. Not exactly. As we'll discuss in much greater detail later, you gained weight by way of a perpetual conflict between *deprivation* and *overindulgence*—neither of which is pleasurable. If you're like most overweight people, you are out of touch with what actually pleases you. In obsessing so much about food, diet, and weight, you have lost your connection with how your body feels and what it really wants.

Chapter 1 | Results Not Typical

The problem, believe it or not, is that you don't enjoy eating *enough*. You think about food more than you actually *experience* food.

Thintuition is excluding every opinion—even your own—about how you should be nourishing yourself, so as to let your body's real needs make themselves heard. It is trusting that your body is inherently wise, capable of knowing and desiring what is best for it. When you say the idea of thintuition sounds too good to be true, what you are really saying is that you don't trust yourself.

And that is hardly surprising. If you've struggled a long time with your weight, you have come to feel that you are not in control of your body. You may even feel it betrays you by blowing up like a balloon the instant you relax your vigilance, punishes you by getting fat when you're just trying to eat like a normal person. (As I'll explain later, your metabolism may indeed be screwed up right now as a result of dieting. The good news is that your body knows how to correct this problem, and will do so when you learn to listen to it better.)

The first reaction of many overweight people is that if they always ate what they really wanted, they'd have ice cream or cheesecake or French fries (or whatever else they're currently forbidding themselves) for breakfast, lunch, and dinner. That's a fantasy born of deprivation. When allowed to express their desires freely, most bodies demand variety. Eat ice cream at every meal for a couple of days, and pretty soon you're likely to lose interest in it and develop a yen for whatever your body is presently missing.

Pregnant women are notorious for the specificity of their food desires. An expectant mother may wake up in the middle of the night with a sudden and imperative yearning for guacamole, want a cheeseburger for breakfast or blueberry pancakes for supper. It is widely (and correctly) assumed that these unusual desires signal some need of the developing fetus or depleted resource in the mother's own system. Pregnant bodies are really no different from other bodies in this respect. The difference is in our attitudes. The expectant mother is *expected* to feel strong desires for specific foods. Because these desires are expected and socially approved, she expresses and fulfills them without inhibition. When you develop your thintuition, you give yourself permission to honor your own needs as a pregnant woman does. If you do this, you will find that your body responds with similar specificity, creating in you the desire for whatever nutrients it presently needs. You don't think, "I need protein." You just ask yourself, "What sounds good?" and find that the answer is something like meatloaf or scrambled eggs.

Look at it another way. How did people figure out what to

eat *before* the advent of modern medical science? Throughout most of human history, people haven't had a clue what proteins, vitamins, or calories even were, much less how many of them were in whatever they were hunting, growing, or gathering. Nevertheless, they managed to nourish themselves just by eating whatever was around that seemed nice to eat. And they didn't get fat! The fact that humanity survived for millennia without scientific knowledge of nutrition is *all* the evidence you need that humans possess inborn intuition about what their bodies need.

When you develop your thintuition, you give yourself permission to honor your own needs.

Doing it

Schwartz observed that thin people tend to enjoy getting hungry and to dislike the sensation of being full. He noted that for many overweight people, the opposite is true. Possibly he underestimated the difficulty this presents when the overweight try to adopt the behaviors of the naturally thin. If you're really going to eat only when hungry, you have to be in touch with what hunger feels like. If you're going to stop when satisfied, you have to be able to recognize that you're satisfied before you feel stuffed. For many overweight people, this is problematic. They are out of touch with the physical signals that tell them when they need to eat and when they need to stop. I will be devoting a whole chapter to this problem later in the book.

For what it's worth, I can testify that I actually did what Schwartz recommends, with spectacular results. And although I know many others who have also succeeded with it as well, I suppose I ought to add the disclaimer that "these results are not typical" of the millions who have read *Diets Don't Work*. If they were, the obesity epidemic would already have abated and the legions of diet experts would be looking for another line of work.

So what's different about me? My story will have amply demonstrated that I'm as capable of failing as the average overweight person, if not more so. I think the only thing that made me different was that, at the time I read Schwartz, I was ready to completely let go of all my previous beliefs. I wasn't just fed up with dieting. I was fed up with *thinking* about diets, fed up with hearing about them and reading about them, deeply and meaningfully disgusted with the whole diet mindset and its many promoters. I wasn't just tired of having a fat body. I was tired of having a fat person's thoughts.

Chapter 1 | Results Not Typical

To succeed with thintuition is to think one simple thought: "I give my body exactly what it needs, no more and no less." But that particular thought is incompatible with nearly every other thought you've ever had about food and weight control. It cannot productively coexist with any of the propaganda of the diet industry, or any of the self-reproaches, admonishments, and intentions you've been filling your head with up 'til now. It's not your body that needs to go on a fast—it's your mind.

That is why I believe that I have something to add to Bob Schwartz's groundbreaking work. I have learned to dispel the thoughts that conflict with my thintuition, to reject them entirely. I hope the following chapters will enable you to do the same.

◆

To succeed with
thintuition is to think
one simple thought:
*"I give my body
exactly what it needs,
no more and no less."*

◆

Chapter 2

How Dieting Makes You Fat

All diets fail in the long run because they have failure built into their design. Diets cannot help but fail because bodies were never meant to engage in repetitive cycles of dramatic weight loss and weight gain. The human body isn't designed to work like that and, just as importantly, neither is the human mind. Human beings were meant to eat in accordance with their body's natural wisdom and so remain as slender as animals in the wild. This eating as our natural instincts dictate is the art and skill of thintuition. It is a form of mindfulness applied to eating. You can succeed *permanently* with it because it is in harmony with your basic nature.

If you're like most dieters, you already know from experience that dieting *can* work in the short run. That's what's so seductive about it. You also know from experience how disappointing it can be in the long run. With each new diet, results seem to come more slowly. And each new weight loss seems to be more short-lived. The pounds come back faster each time you go off a diet and, if your results are typical, you eventually find that you weigh more than you did when you started.

It's not your imagination and it's not your fault. This predictable failure is built in to both human physiology and human psychology. You are failing because what you are attempting to do is in direct conflict with your basic nature.

Dieting messes up your metabolism

Let's quickly review what you already know. Food supplies energy. What you don't convert to energy before the next meal gets stored for later use as fat. If you've got a lot of fat, you're storing more potential energy than you're ever going to need. So it seems perfectly logical to try to correct the problem by taking in less than you need at the moment, obliging your body to burn what it has previously stored. That's how the whole idea of dieting got started.

Unfortunately, it's a bit more complicated than that. You see, for most of human history, getting enough food has been a big hassle. Food tended to arrive by fits and starts. If you lived by hunting, you killed a big animal now and then, and ate the whole thing before it spoiled, knowing it could be days or weeks before you managed to kill another one and eat again. If you lived by farming, there was loads to eat at harvest time and you stuffed yourself then, knowing that the pickings would be slim all winter.

The human body, in its wisdom, adapted by slowing down its energy demands (metabolism) whenever food was scarce. When it wasn't getting calories, it figured there were no calories to be had and learned to get along on fewer of them. In times of scarcity, everyone's body slowed down, rationing the potential energy that had previously been stored. The constant abundance of food most people in the developed world currently enjoy is something that the human body has only encountered relatively recently in its evolution. If this abundance had always been the norm, you can be sure that the body would have adapted itself to cope with excessive—rather than inadequate—quantities of food. People would be able to eat as much food as they wanted without ever getting fat.

When you overeat, your body does not question why you are giving it more food than it needs. It just knows instinctively that too much eating means that the times are good. And so, being provident, it holds on to the excess food you offer it as a hedge against future hard times. That is its wisdom. If you ever did find yourself hard pressed to find food, you'd be glad of the fat it has stored.

Similarly, when you eat too little, your body assumes there's no food to be had. From the body's point of view, dieting means scarcity, impending starvation. The body doesn't know that all you want to do is look good on the beach. As far as it can tell, the harvest has failed and the buffaloes have all run away. No telling where the next meal is coming from, so better slow down and conserve energy. When you don't eat enough, your body's sole concern is to keep you alive until the famine is over. The more frequently these "famines" come, the quicker on the uptake your body becomes. If you diet several times a year, your body figures you're living in Ethiopia. That's why you've got such a slow metabolism. It's also why your body hangs on for dear life to whatever extra calories you consume when you eventually go off the diet. It is actually true that you can't eat as much as normal people eat without getting fat. You're not just imagining this. Habitual dieters are literally *training* their bodies to live on fewer and fewer calories, and to store food more efficiently as fat.

You have probably heard that it takes more calories to sustain muscle than to sustain fat. This is true. When you diet, the weight you lose is composed of water, fat, and muscle. When you go off the diet, the weight you regain is mostly fat and water. So with every diet you are changing your fat-to-lean ratio for the worse. That means you need fewer calories to maintain your current weight than you would need if you weighed the same but had never dieted. This is another reason why the more you diet, the less you can eat without getting fat.

If you understand your body's logic, you will also be able to see what you need to do to correct your metabolic problem. You have to send your body the message that you are not, after all, going through a famine or anticipating one any time soon. You do this by eating enough—and no more than enough—every time you are hungry. To your body, enough right now means that food is readily available. No more than enough means that you expect food to be in good supply for the foreseeable future and don't need to stockpile. When it gets this message consistently, your body becomes less cautious about expending energy. Your metabolism speeds up. Even if you're not exercising much, you feel more energetic, more alert and alive, just sitting still.

Dieting exaggerates your interest in food

It stands to reason that what occupies our attention day and night will tend to dominate our lives. Most diets require us to make special arrangements for our eating. You may have to buy different foods for yourself than you buy for the other members of your household, and you may have to prepare your food in a special way. You have to interrogate your server before ordering in a restaurant and read the fine print on every package before putting it in your grocery cart. You probably also have to count something—calories, carbs, fat grams, or "winning points." All of these activities lead you to think about food more than you otherwise would. All this thinking you do about food is what makes you different from a thin person.

In a study conducted by Ancel Keys, Ph.D., during the Korean War, a group of naturally thin male volunteers were put on a strict diet. Being of normal weight at the outset, they were not in the habit of giving much thought to food. But soon after the experiment commenced, food became the main topic of their every conversation. They read about it. They daydreamed about it. Halfway through the experiment, thirteen of them expressed the intention of becoming professional cooks! For most of them, the obsession with food continued long after the experiment ended and they were allowed to return to normal eating. Many reported insistent cravings for specific foods—cravings they'd never experienced before the diet. Many also reported that they often felt driven to eat more than they believed they really needed and had trouble noticing when they were getting full or stopping

Chapter 2 | How Dieting Makes You Fat

themselves when they did notice. Some developed persistent weight problems.

In another study done at the University of Toronto in 1975, psychologists C. Peter Herman and Deborah Mack served their experimental subjects with milkshakes, then brought in ice cream and told them they could eat as much of it as they wanted. The subjects were divided into three groups. Group One received two servings of milkshake before the ice cream appeared. Group Two received just one milkshake, and Group Three got no milkshake at all. When the experiment was performed on people who had never dieted, the researchers got the results they were expecting. The less milkshake the subjects had previously consumed, the more ice cream they ate. You're probably wondering why they had to do a scientific experiment to discover something so obvious, right?

Well, here's the interesting part. When the experiment was repeated with frequent dieters for subjects, the results were exactly the opposite. The group that had been given two milkshakes at the start of the test actually ate the *most* ice cream.

For a naturally thin person, to stop eating when satisfied requires no special will power. The thought of eating simply vanishes as soon as hunger ceases. But to resist the cravings induced by dieting requires a tremendous struggle, because the thought of a particular food often refuses to go away until that food is actually eaten. Even if you don't give in to the craving, resisting its incessant prompting requires a huge expenditure of mental energy. You become mentally and emotionally exhausted and, in your fatigue, find it harder and harder to remain in control. And if you give in to the craving, you may find yourself eating a ridiculous quantity of the "forbidden" food, gorging yourself till you feel almost sick.

Believe it or not, this highly annoying fact is also an expression of the body's natural wisdom. A person who is starving doesn't especially feel like plowing a field, hunting a mastodon, or scaling a tree to get a banana. In order to motivate someone whose energy is low to go to the trouble of obtaining food, the human organism responds to what it perceives as potential starvation by making thoughts of food more compelling. The more you resist, the more your body insists. "Will power" only exacerbates the problem. Your body insists louder because you don't seem to be listening. Your cravings may vastly exceed any real physical need because your body has gone into emergency mode. By dieting, you have confused it into believing it is starving. That's how it interprets rapid weight loss and repeatedly unsatisfied hunger. When a body in starvation mode finally gets what it has been wanting, it responds as if preparing to survive the next Ice Age.

Admittedly, it's hard to see the craving for something like cheese curls as an expression of natural wisdom. We often crave foods that have little to offer nutritionally, foods we could perfectly well do without for the rest of our lives. Later we'll discuss the emotional component of some of these irrational cravings. For now, the point I want you to get is that naturally thin people don't have them. They eat what they desire without passing judgment on their desire, and as a result they are able to desire and eat in moderation. They may eat foods of dubious nutritional value, but they don't crave or binge on these foods. A desire that is *satisfied* when it arises does not escalate into a craving.

Dieting diminishes your confidence

When we diet, we are attempting to impose conscious control on a process that was designed to occur automatically and instinctively. That's what we mean by "will power." If you succeed at all, it's at the expense of a tremendous inner struggle that very few people are able to sustain year in and year out. Trying to do what your body and mind were never designed to do sets you up for eventual failure. These repeated failures can be devastating to the self-esteem of the dieter.

Our temporary successes with dieting only make matters worse. Each time you diet down to your goal weight, you feel triumphant about all the temptations you managed to resist along the way. You have managed to accomplish something very difficult, against tremendous odds. People admire you for your tenacity, and you admire yourself. But this sense of triumph sets you up to lose confidence as soon as you start to regain the weight. If getting thin means you are a paragon of self-discipline, getting fat again must mean that you are undisciplined, self-indulgent, and out of control. When you yo-yo diet, your self-confidence fluctuates in inverse proportion to your weight.

The phenomenon can be especially perplexing to the many overweight people who are confident, disciplined, and assertive in other aspects of their lives. You may have no trouble at all making and keeping conscious resolutions that have nothing to do with food. When you resolve to do things like limiting your credit card spending, returning phone calls promptly, folding the laundry as soon as it comes out of the dryer, or reading to your child every night, you are able to follow through consistently. Your conscious intentions lead reliably to desired actions and you feel like you are in control of yourself—except when it comes to your weight. If you're like most dieters, you take this very personally. The fact that the majority of dieters go on secret binges doesn't enter into your consideration at the moment you are hating yourself for the latest food fest. Your failure feels unique and entirely personal, the expression of some fatal flaw in your character. You may even have labeled yourself a "food addict."

In an effort to shore up your wobbly self-esteem, you may then start looking for external excuses. The idea that your problem might be genetic has tremendous appeal, because your genes are obviously not your fault. Yet attributing the problem to a factor entirely outside your control leads to further feelings of helplessness. If the cause is really genetic, there's not a damn thing you can do about it.

The shame that overweight people feel is all the more cruel because many of them have shed literally thousands of pounds of fat in their repeated attempts to diet. If you have managed to lose weight by dieting, you have tremendous will power—far more than the average thin person. It is not that you lack self-discipline. It's that you have been applying discipline to the wrong activity.

In the Ancel Keys study, many of the participants developed serious psychological problems. They became anxious, withdrawn, and depressed. Their concentration and their interest in the world around them declined. Many also became extremely critical of their own bodies. Recall that none of these men was overweight at the time the diet began. Despite the fact that their bodies were normal to begin with, and becoming thinner, some of them began, for the first time in their lives, to perceive themselves as fat. They developed all sorts of new complaints about the size and shape of their bodies. For just as dieting makes you think too much about food, it also leads to thinking too much about how you look.

This is particularly painful in a society that equates beauty with thinness. On any given day, you are bombarded with countless direct and subliminal advertising messages telling you that fat is unattractive and defeatist, and that people who are fat are more likely to be failures in their social, sexual, and professional lives. The diet industry wants you to feel bad about being fat. What else but self-loathing would drive you to eat their unappealing foods, experiment with potentially dangerous supplements, or adopt goofy regimens for which there is no scientific support?

This is not to say that being obese is good. If you are carrying a significant amount of excess weight, losing it will likely make you healthier and happier. But dieting often leads to an excessive focus on weight, which comes to seem like the sole cause of any and every problem and disappointment. If we lose a close relationship or suffer a career setback, we tend to blame our weight. Conversely, we may develop unrealistic ideas about how great our lives would be if we could just get thin. These exaggerated hopes and fears about fat contribute to the extreme emotional ups and downs that accompany yo-yo dieting.

It's not that you lack self-discipline. It's that you have been applying discipline to the wrong activity.

Dieting encourages you to abdicate your personal power

The premise of thintuition is that you, and you alone, are the ultimate authority on what, when, and how much you should eat. Nobody else knows if you are hungry. Nobody else knows what nutrients your body needs at this particular moment. This information comes from your own body, and the only way to know it is to pay attention to what your body is telling you.

When you diet, you are giving away this natural authority to someone else. You are looking outside yourself for the answers. It doesn't really matter whether the advice you're following is good or bad, whether it's based on sound scientific research or the kooky belief system of some formerly fat celebrity. From the perspective of thintuition, even *good* advice is *bad* for you because, in taking it, you are basing your behavior on abstract thoughts about food and eating rather than the actual experience of hunger and satisfaction.

Take for example the idea that you shouldn't skip breakfast. The reasoning behind this idea seems to make a lot of sense. So maybe you don't feel hungry when you first wake up, but you dutifully consume a "sensible" breakfast: half a grapefruit, a poached egg, and a slice of whole wheat toast. If your body actually needed these foods at this time, you would have woken up hungry for them. Indisputably sensible as this meal might be, to eat it at this moment is to overeat. Your eating is motivated by an abstract idea ("Breakfast is good for me") rather than by physical hunger.

The same goes for the apparently sensible idea of portion control. Since overeating makes you fat, it seems perfectly logical to measure and limit portion size. But the idea that six ounces of chicken is an appropriate portion is entirely irrelevant to your body's needs. Six ounces of chicken might have been too much yesterday; it might be too little tomorrow. Depends on how hungry you are. Until you're actually eating it, you don't know how much chicken you need. Your body will tell you by ceasing to send hunger signals when it's had enough.

Chapter 2 | How Dieting Makes You Fat

In following a diet, most of us tend to internalize its author as our personal judge. The process is especially blatant when restaurants tout certain menu items as "doctor approved." Who cares if Dr. So and So approves of you? Approval never made anyone thin.

In dieting, we don't just surrender our personal power to the diet "experts," we endow foods themselves with the power to make us thin or fat. If you're following a low-fat regime, you believe that a cheese omelet and three strips of bacon for breakfast will make you fat, while cereal with fruit will make you thin. If you're following a low-carb regime, you believe the opposite. Nutrition moderates often criticize such diets on the grounds that they lead people to eliminate foods that are good for them. Equally dangerous to the dieter is the subconscious magical belief that the "good" foods on a diet—the ones you're allowed to eat in unlimited quantities—will somehow cause weight loss. It is as if, by eating Lean Cuisine, we believe we are ingesting the quality of leanness.

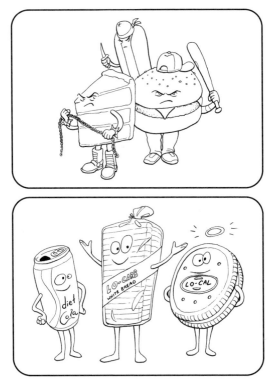

"bad" foods and "good" foods

We endow foods themselves with the power to make us thin or fat.

When we label certain foods as "good" or "bad" we subtly endow them with the power to make *us* good or bad. You really want a cheeseburger, but instead you order a green salad with low-fat dressing on the side. What a good girl or boy you are! Your lunch companions must be basking in the glow of your halo. Or, you knew you shouldn't have that chocolate cake, but you couldn't resist the temptation. Naughty, naughty! Our moralizing about food has become so extreme that people are starting to treat the selling of fast food as the moral equivalent of making napalm or nerve gas. Your conscience has better things to do than to pass judgment on everything you put in your stomach. The contents of your lunch box are not the content of your character.

How did you decide what you should weigh in the first place? If your notion of your ideal weight came from your doctor, the Body Mass Index, or the professed weight of your favorite supermodel, you are giving the power to decide what's good for you to someone else. That is not necessarily to say that you're trying to weigh too little. (When I began to practice thintuition, I eventually stabilized at a much lower

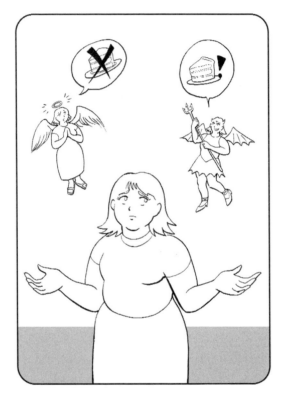

"Will eating devil's food cake
make me a bad person?"

Chapter 2 | How Dieting Makes You Fat

weight than I'd been expecting.) The issue is the motivation behind the goal, not the goal itself. You have achieved your personal best when the size of your body is no longer an obstacle to anything you want in life, and when you can maintain your desired size without obsessing about it. The right weight for you is the weight that *feels* great. You can't know what it is by consulting a chart or comparing yourself to other people.

Thintuition is a process of reconnecting with your own physical experience. To begin practicing it requires a leap of faith, for dieting has trained you to distrust your body and your choices. If every time you've stopped dieting in the past you've ended up overeating and putting on weight, you may have come to believe that this is your natural inclination. In fact, it is an *unnatural* inclination induced by the emotional and metabolic stress of rebound dieting. You cannot correct by dieting a problem that is *caused* by dieting. When you make a firm and lasting commitment to stop doing this to yourself, your metabolism will gradually self-correct and your cravings will abate. Bodies are very smart.

◆

You have achieved
your personal best
when the size of your
body is no longer
an obstacle to anything
you want in life.

◆

Chapter 3
The Overfed Head

Imagine what it would be like if all the citizens of the greatest and most powerful nation in the world were suddenly afflicted by a mysterious and irresistible compulsion to alternate between cycles of self-inflicted food deprivation and ravenous eating, until they became as bloated as balloons. Imagine each person slowly succumbing to diseases, breathlessness, organ failure, humiliation, fear, confusion, panic, and disorientation—and death.

Thankfully, we're not quite there yet. But we're getting there fast because, as a nation, we are being more and more conditioned to accept misleading explanations of and counterproductive solutions to our weight problems. Despite the mass of empirical evidence that dieting makes matters worse, we continue to be bombarded with the mythology that this or that variation on dieting is different from all others, and will solve our problem once and for all.

Where does all this diet mythology come from? Most of it

wasn't around in your grandmother's day. Although interest in dieting dates back to the nineteenth century, it didn't have widespread impact until recently, because the *commercial* possibilities inherent in making people obsessive about food and weight hadn't been recognized and exploited. Both the problem of overweight and our obsession with the problem have *escalated* in proportion to the growth of information and communication technology. This is no coincidence.

It was quite possible, one hundred years ago, to live a happy, active and productive life without being affected in any significant way by the power of advertising. But since those relatively innocent times, the situation has changed out of all recognition. The modern advertising industry has the ability to reach every man, woman, and child in this country, and to infiltrate your consciousness morning, noon, and night. And the impact of advertising messages has become infinitely more powerful and seductive than it was even forty years ago. Modern advertising techniques are able to target specifically defined groups with the lethal accuracy of a sniper's bullet.

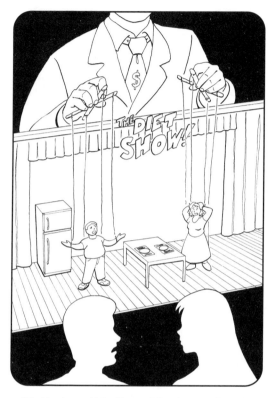

"Betty, I can't believe this show takes in
$40 billion a year."

To get an idea of the scope of the problem, watch television for two or three hours and make a note of every single message you receive about food, body and weight. You will discover how repetitively you are inundated with the following impressions:

- People with thin, shapely bodies are happy, healthy, and desirable.
- Certain foods make you fat.
- Certain foods cause health problems.
- Certain foods make you thin.
- Certain foods can prevent disease.
- The foods that make you fat are delicious.
- Eating is fun.
- Special occasions require special foods.
- Large quantities of food are a bargain.
- Certain foods give you indigestion, but you can remedy this by taking medicine.
- You can lose weight rapidly by:
    - a) enrolling in a program
    - b) joining a gym
    - c) buying a book
    - d) eating special foods
    - e) taking a drug or diet supplement
    - f) having a gastric bypass operation

In other words, during a single evening of television viewing, you are repeatedly enticed to eat whether hungry or not while being reminded constantly that the resulting fat is unhealthy and unattractive. Torn by these conflicting influences, you are offered a variety of products and services that promise to resolve the conflict.

Taken as a whole, the messages you absorb from the culture express a schizophrenic sort of consumerism. You are exhorted to consume food for all sorts of reasons besides hunger, and then to consume various other products (including foods) to undo the lamentable results. The only consistent element in these otherwise contradictory propositions is that what you need to lose weight lies *outside* of yourself and has to be purchased.

If this were a conscious conspiracy to make Americans fat and unhappy, you'd have to admire its brilliance. But it's not a conspiracy. It's just what happens when a lot of different industries and professions—many of them quite well-intentioned—go about the business of making a buck. Your problem is their opportunity. It is a basic fact of economic life that when profit can be made from a problem, those who profit have a natural stake in its continuation. A *permanent* solution would eventually eliminate its very reason for existence. From a business point of view, the ideal solution is one that subtly exacerbates the customer's problem, leading to further demand.

Imagine for a moment what would happen if scientists were to discover a cheap and easily produced substitute for gasoline. Such a discovery would certainly revolutionize the world as we know it, just as the invention of the internal combustion engine made the horse and carriage obsolete within a couple of decades. But what would be the effect of such a discovery on the multi-billion-dollar oil industry? Those whose fabulous wealth is derived from our dependence on petroleum obviously could not be expected to rejoice over the development of a cheap and renewable source of energy. To invest in perpetuating the problem is a much safer bet than investing in its solution.

The industrial equivalent of diets is *planned obsolescence,* where a product is designed to fail or wear out quickly so that you will go out and buy a new one. The short-term success followed by long-term failure that is built in to dieting ensures that you will trade in last year's diet for a newer model as soon as the pounds return. The cycle can continue profitably so long as customers blame themselves—rather than the product—for the transience of the benefits.

After reading the last chapter, you may be thoroughly convinced that dieting is not only useless, but actively harmful. You suspected so all along, didn't you? Yet despite the wealth of evidence that this is so, most people have a lot of trouble resisting the allure of diet mythology. This is due partly to the sheer volume of diet propaganda circulating in the culture. But it is also because, whether true or not, diet mythology can be very persuasive. So let's examine some of the ways it sucks you in.

The appeal of scientific authority

The medical profession over the years has lent its authority and prestige to dieting as a means of losing weight. The reasons for this are obvious. Doctors are seeing more and more people whose health and quality of life are being seriously jeopardized because they are overweight or obese. The medical profession knows better than we do that excess weight increases the risk of potentially fatal or crippling conditions that afflict millions of Americans every year. You yourself are probably familiar with these frightening statistics because we are constantly being reminded of them in the media.

While most doctors agree that obesity is medically dangerous, that is pretty much the only fact about which they have achieved scientific consensus. For every diet approach backed by a bestselling M.D., you will find a host of other physicians telling you that it's scientifically unfounded at best, and possibly downright dangerous. Some doctors specialize in gastric bypass operations. Others recommend against them. Doctors are not even in perfect accord about what you should weigh in the first place. Some will say that an extra twenty pounds is a medical issue that ought to be addressed, while others will assert that the effects of frequently losing and regaining that twenty pounds are actually more detrimental than carrying the extra weight consistently. If scientific knowledge is defined as those facts about which scientists have achieved overwhelming consensus based on consistent experimental data, it must be admitted that there is very little scientific knowledge about weight control.

Most dieters know from bitter experience that the results of dieting are temporary at best, and that weight loss becomes more difficult with each new diet. Between bouts of self-reproach, intelligent dieters quite reasonably suspect that there is some physiological reason for this that science might eventually explain. When a new diet, based on some new scientific—or pseudo-scientific—principle arrives on the scene, it is natural to hope that the magic formula has finally been discovered. Diets that target certain food types or food combinations while promising that you can eat unlimited amounts of other food types have particular appeal because they absolve the dieter of responsibility for previous failures. Just as you suspected, the problem is not that you eat too much. It's that until now, nobody realized that certain foods or food combinations are more likely to be converted to fat. Now that the secret has finally been revealed, you'll be able to eat as much as you want and stay slim.

In our fascination with the intricacy of these theories, it's very easy to lose sight of the big picture. Throughout most of human history, people have eaten the full variety of foods available to them, naively combining them on the basis of what tastes good: bread and butter, beans and rice, pancakes and syrup, meat and potatoes, crackers and cheese. If this procedure really caused people to get fat, the epidemic of obesity we're now seeing would not be a new phenomenon. Similarly, many of the artificial substitutes for foods that are now considered fattening are of very recent invention. If using these substitutes were truly helpful to weight control, you would expect Americans to be getting *thinner* instead of *fatter.* Or what about the theory of genetic predisposition to fat? If that is truly the explanation, why do so many fat people have *skinny* ancestors?

The allure of quick and dramatic results

Dieting often *does* work—in the short term. You have probably achieved rapid and substantial weight loss on previous diets, and you remember how great you felt about that success. So when you feel a pressing need to lose weight quickly—to fit into your summer clothes or look good for some special occasion—the prospect of quick results can be extremely enticing. On any given day that you conceive this desire, you can turn on the television or open a magazine and read stories of people who have achieved it on some sort of diet.

Some of this advertising is outright deceptive. For example, in some ads, the models were photographed for the "after" picture *first,* then paid to put on weight for the "before" picture. In other cases, both photos are taken on the same day, the apparent weight loss being achieved through a combination of make-up, lighting, and posture. But even when the weight loss depicted in such ads is genuine, you are being subtly misled to generalize from the atypical experience of a few. They tell you about isolated individuals who have met—and maybe even maintained—their goal weight, rather than providing you with statistics about the *average* amount of weight lost by participants in a program and the *average* length of time this weight loss is maintained.

Would you sign on for a diet program if you knew for sure that a dramatic weight loss would inevitably be followed by an even more dramatic weight *gain*? Or if you knew that the weight loss could be maintained, but only by following the diet strictly for the rest of your life? Your own experience will confirm that these are the actual results of dieting. Yet the diet ads play on a hope that springs eternal, leading the dieter to fall again and again for the con that all previous diets were simply the wrong diet, and that with the right diet, everything will be different.

Dieting reminds me of the ancient myth of Sisyphus, who was condemned by the gods to spend all eternity rolling a stone up a hill, only to watch it roll down again once he'd pushed it to the top. You are living the same myth so long as you allow yourself to be persuaded that your latest diet is the last one you'll ever have to push up the hill.

Misery loves company

If dieting is a delusion, it is at least a *mass* delusion. How do you face reality when everyone around you is busy perpetuating the lunacy of diet mythology?

We are socially rewarded for doing what everyone else is doing, thinking what everyone else is thinking, discussing

The Overfed Head

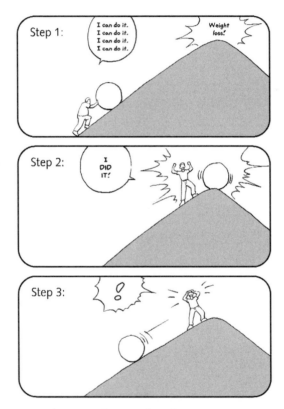

. . . and repeat four to five times per year.

what everyone else is discussing. In contemporary America, dieting is second only to the weather as a universal topic of conversation. When you dine out with friends, they don't just order, they *editorialize* about what they are ordering. Almost everyone these days has a food theory. If you take the view that food is just fuel, you won't have much to contribute to the conversation. (When was the last time you heard people discussing their choices at the gas pump?)

Dieting also creates a lot of drama. While on a diet, you can regale friends, family, and co-workers with a blow-by-blow account of your progress, your triumphs and setbacks, how easy or difficult you are finding it. As the weight comes off, people notice and congratulate you. Run into someone you haven't seen in a while and the first comment you hear is how much thinner you look. When you slim down, you get loads of praise for both your appearance and the effort you've made. You also get to hold forth as a diet expert, explaining how you did it and exhorting your overweight friends to take the same approach. Fluctuating weight gets you a lot of attention.

You may even have relationships that are based entirely on your struggle to lose weight—perhaps a support group formed through your diet or fitness center. The warm encouragement and commiseration you receive from these people may depend to some extent on your remaining in the same boat with them. You may also have adopted your diet coach or trainer as a sort of mentor—a friendly parent figure whom you seek to please with your weekly weigh-ins and your adherence to their advice.

You can gauge how much social satisfaction you obtain from dieting by asking yourself, "How much do I talk to others about my diet when I am dieting?" If it's a lot, social reinforcement may be luring you back into diet after diet, against your better judgment. Consider how your relationships might change if your weight were to stabilize in the normal range and cease to be a preoccupation. What would you talk about instead?

Partial truths

The overall falsehood of diet mythology is peppered with a few truths about nutrition, exercise, and general health. For example, it is true that some foods provide better nourishment than other foods. It is also true that if you exercise regularly, you are likely to look and feel better and to be happier with your body. These facts are undeniable. They just *don't* happen to be especially relevant to the question of weight control.

Chapter 3 | The Overfed Head

If exercise were the key to weight control, you would expect to see a correlation between the physical demands of a person's job and their body weight. Construction workers, furniture movers, janitors, and kindergarten teachers would tend to be thinner, on the whole, than accountants, writers, and computer programmers. This is obviously not the case. You find plenty of heavy people in active occupations, and plenty of skinny people with sedentary jobs.

Exercise does burn calories, but not that many. You'd have to walk for an hour to burn off a cookie. Its real benefits to weight control are less direct. Regular exercise accelerates the resting metabolism and increases muscle mass, both of which optimize the efficiency with which you burn calories all day. It reduces stress and gives a feeling of overall well-being, which can be a help if you tend to overeat when nervous or unhappy. People who exercise also tend to like their bodies more, even if they're overweight. Personally, I love to work out, and have even taught exercise classes. So don't think I'm knocking it when I say that reliance on exercise for weight control is an expression of the diet mentality that's keeping you overweight.

The problem lies in making a mental connection between exercise and eating. After a strenuous workout, chronic dieters tell themselves that they get to eat more, or *need* to eat more. It may or may not be true that you are hungrier after exercise, but that's not the point. The point is that eating more is your conscious or unconscious *objective.* You are trying to need more food in order to justify eating it. Why? If you are trying to increase your hunger, you must have some reason other than hunger for wanting food in the first place. That desire for food in the absence of *need* for food is what distinguishes you from a naturally thin person. When overweight people exercise in order to justify eating, they tend to exaggerate the hunger they've worked up and to overeat. I wholeheartedly encourage you to exercise if that's what you feel like doing. But to succeed with thintuition, you will need to make a complete conceptual separation between exercise and eating.

The idea that some foods are better than others *from a nutritional standpoint* is obviously true. Making good nutritional choices will certainly contribute to your health, but this will *not* make you thin. You can get very fat on a balanced, healthy diet. You can also stay slim eating nothing but junk food. What makes you fat or thin is not *what* you eat, but *why* you are eating. To eat for *any* reason other than hunger will cause you to put on weight. That fact is no less true if you are eating to get your minimum daily requirement of some nutrient.

The trouble with being nutritionally conscious is that it tends to exaggerate the power and importance of food. We are told to avoid certain foods because they cause diseases and to consume other foods because they have the power to prevent diseases. It's the latter proposition that makes the biggest impression on the overfed mind. Doctors and nutrition experts say to eat more fiber, or eat more fruits and vegetables, or eat more foods rich in antioxidants. On an unconscious level, the message absorbed by an overweight person is simply *"eat more."* Like exercise, nutrition becomes our mental justification for overeating.

Let's get real. When was the last time you saw an American afflicted with scurvy or beriberi? Malnutrition is very low on the list of health risks you face, especially if you're overweight. When you learn to tune into your body's promptings, you will find yourself drawn to the foods it *actually* needs—which may or may not resemble your current theory about what it needs. If you continue to believe you require nutrients that you're not actually getting hungry for, take a daily multivitamin and stop worrying about it. For an overweight person, excessive thinking about food presents a far greater health risk than not eating enough oat bran.

It is theorized that some foods may cause allergies or addictions, leading us to crave them when we actually should be avoiding them. Yet research has shown that craving is a predictable result of dieting alone. Imbalances that have arisen from dieting usually correct themselves over time when you start to satisfy your natural food preferences and eat moderately. Certainly if you have been diagnosed with a specific allergy or a condition such as diabetes, you should heed your doctor's recommendations as to what foods are off limits. You can still follow your thintuition by choosing to eat what you like best from the list of foods that are safe for you.

Making good nutritional choices will certainly contribute to your health, but this will not make you thin.

To practice thintuition is to regard your natural inclinations as the sole and absolute authority on what, when, and how much to eat. All other theories are incompatible with it. This is not just because so many of these theories are false and unproductive. From the standpoint of thintuition, even a well-founded theory that is working well for other dieters is unhelpful. Reliance on *any* external authority—even a very smart one—diverts your attention from your own experience. It leads you to make food choices based on abstract ideas rather than your natural instincts.

Chapter 3 | The Overfed Head

If your body is overweight, your head is overfed. All the thinking you do about food and weight has led to an unhealthy obsession, an exaggeration of food's power to help or harm you. It's your head—not your body—that needs to be on a diet. As once you resisted cheesecake and potato chips, you now need to learn to resist the all-you-can-think buffet of food and diet information, no matter how enticing you find some of the items on offer.

The decision to practice thintuition entails some initial loss. You've invested a lot of time and energy in acquiring masses of information that you will now need to disregard. It can be painful to admit that all this past effort was of no avail. It can also be scary. All that information you've acquired has been subconsciously training you to distrust your own instincts. You have been told again and again that, left to your own devices, you will make the wrong choices. Those extra pounds you're carrying seem to prove it. In the next chapter we'll explore some of the psychological factors that have led you to make poor choices in the past, and talk about how to reestablish self-trust.

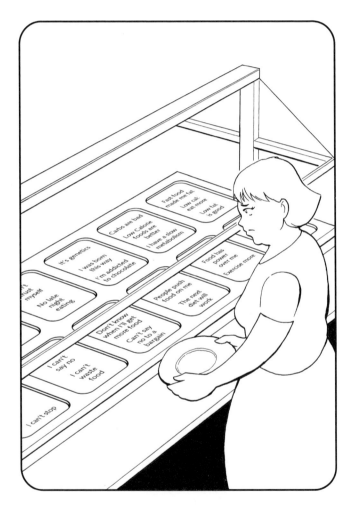

"I think I'll have the cheesecake instead."

◆

To practice thintuition is to regard your natural inclinations as the sole and absolute authority on what, when, and how much to eat.

◆

Chapter 4

Inaccurate Eating

Ina recent internet survey, participants were asked to choose the primary reason why so many Americans are overweight. The multiple choices offered included factors such as metabolism, genetic predisposition, lack of exercise, and specific food choices. Overeating was not even listed as one of the options. It seems the current trend in the U.S. is to blame overweight on anything and everything *but* the actual cause.

Face it: if you weigh more than you should, you are eating more food than your body needs. The idea is unpopular partly because it places the responsibility for excess pounds on the person carrying them. How can you be responsible for what you can't seem to control, no matter how hard you try? The issue is further complicated by the fact that many overweight people eat no more than thin people. If your metabolism has gotten confused by frequent dieting, it may literally be true that you can't eat what you consider to be a "normal" amount without gaining weight. The condition is correctable, but for the moment, you are stuck with its unhappy consequences. The prospect of having to eat like a bird all the time to get thin lends tremendous appeal to any diet that permits unlimited quantities of certain foods.

So what *is* the right amount to eat? You will remain confused about this so long as you are trying to conform to some external standard. Comparing what you eat to what other people eat, to what your favorite restaurant considers an appropriate portion size, or to some objective measure such as daily calories, fat grams, carbs, etc., leads to inaccurate eating. The external standard means nothing to your body. Attempt to conform to it and you will end up eating too much or too little. Inaccuracy in either direction is what confuses your metabolism.

The right amount to eat is determined *solely* by your hunger. What you eat when truly hungry will not make you fat, because hunger is a sign that your body is ready to convert food to energy. Conversely, anything you eat when not truly hungry will get stored as fat, because that's how your body handles nourishment that it can't immediately use. Your diet may "permit" or even require you to eat a seemingly nonfattening snack such as an apple in the middle of the afternoon. If you're not actually hungry at snack time, that apple is contributing to the problem, not the solution.

The Overfed Head

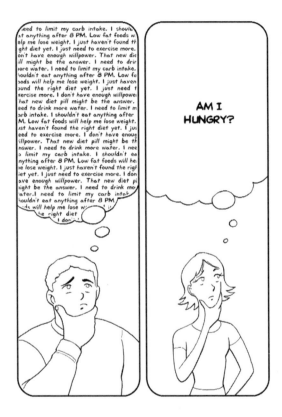

On the other hand, if you *are* very hungry and what you want is apple pie, there is no reason to deny yourself.

While the notion of harmless apple pie is immensely appealing, part of you is probably regarding it as dangerous. In the past you've gone overboard on the foods that you like best. Thintuition is a freedom you're afraid you might abuse. That's a legitimate worry if you're being driven to eat by motives other than hunger. And right now you are. If you didn't eat for reasons other than hunger, you would not have become overweight in the first place.

In *Diets Don't Work,* Bob Schwartz used the term "emotional eating" to cover all impulses we have to eat when we don't physically need to. Some of these motives have subsequently gotten a lot of airplay. On talk shows you will hear from people who have been sexually abused and went on to get fat as an unconscious defense against unwanted sexual attention. You hear about people who learned to comfort themselves with food when feeling neglected as children, about people who turn to food for relief when feeling stressed, about people who eat in defiance of an overly controlling parent or partner. Maybe you identify with some of these stories.

It's true that some people are driven to overeat by the kind of deep-seated emotional issues that require therapeutic support. But there are many other motives for overeating that are not dramatic enough to provide fodder for talk shows. Let's consider some examples.

- Stan travels frequently on business. While the airlines used to provide meals on almost every flight, as a cost-cutting measure they've now gotten miserly with food. Add frequent delays to the equation and there's a real possibility you might find yourself stuck in the air for hours with nothing to eat but a packet of peanuts. To prepare for this eventuality, Stan takes the precaution of downing a couple of slices of pizza just before boarding any flight. He adopts the same strategy before going into a meeting that he expects to run long, or starting a workday that he expects to be very busy. Unexpected hunger is a hassle he doesn't want to have to deal with, so he eats more than his fill at the times when it's convenient for him to eat.

- Jessica attends an aerobics class right after work, three evenings a week. Although she's not especially hungry when she leaves the office, she's afraid she'll run out of energy before the class is over, so she grabs an energy bar. After class, she often treats herself to a big dinner, figuring she needs the extra sustenance. Any time her energy is running low, Jessica assumes she needs to eat.

- When she was a child, Emily was a very picky eater. Every family dinner seemed to turn into a major struggle with her parents, who spent the whole meal trying to coax, cajole, or threaten her into cleaning her plate. Her inner conflicts around food and autonomy have led to a lifetime of yo-yo dieting. Her weight fluctuates between borderline obese and fashion model skinny.

- As a child, Emily's older sister Amy came to define herself in contrast to her "problem child" sister by dutifully eating whatever was put before her. Her parents often praised her for this and exhorted Emily to be more like her. As an adult, Amy persists in her pattern of "sensible" eating, dutifully consuming three square meals a day whether she wants them or not. For years her weight has remained stable. Though she weighs about thirty pounds more than she wants to, she believes it is much saner to resign herself to being moderately overweight than to fluctuate between extremes like her sister.

- As a cost accountant, George is vigilant about avoiding waste. At any function where food is served, he'll eat whether hungry or not, for he figures that every free meal is an offset to his own food budget. For the same reason, he favors all-you-can eat restaurants, making two or three trips to the buffet table to ensure that he gets his money's worth. Rather than waste money by throwing food away, he will force himself to finish the leftovers in his fridge before they spoil.

- Dimitri's strong libido attracted Katrina when she first married him, but after their first few months together, it began to exhaust her. Her own sex drive was much lower, and she didn't feel adequate to meeting his needs. As if to compensate for this perceived failure, she began to cook big and elaborate meals. Sated by her heavy cooking, Dimitri often dozed on the couch after dinner, and made fewer sexual advances. Perhaps she was also becoming less desirable to him as she put on weight. Without ever adopting this as a conscious plan, Katrina had discovered that their mutual appetite for food could smooth over the disparity in their sexual appetites.

- For Erica, food is an expression of her sensuality and her love of life. She's a fantastic cook and loves to give dinner parties. An avid reader of restaurant reviews, she enjoys sampling exotic ethnic cuisines and the work of fashionable chefs. Eating is also one of the chief pleasures of travel for her, and the presence of a renowned restaurant is reason enough to place an out-of-the-way town on her itinerary. A "seize-the-day" eater, she tends to regard each meal as a unique and wonderful experience that won't come again, a slice of life that she insists on living to the fullest.

- Billy has been suffering from bouts of homesickness ever since he moved to New York from his native Alabama. When he's feeling depressed by the physical coldness of the climate and the emotional coldness of the big city, he indulges in food nostalgia. A feast of all his down-home favorites puts him back in touch with his Southern roots and gives him a warm fuzzy feeling.

- Jeff's work as a labor mediator is very stressful. He spends a lot of time around angry, argumentative people, and needs to be a voice of calm and reason. When he's feeling edgy, he finds that it helps to eat a lot of heavy carbohydrates. A couple of donuts for breakfast or a big plate of pasta for lunch seems to dull the rough edges, slow down his racing mind, and make him feel calmer.

• Myra, the mother of five small children, is bewildered by the forty pounds she's gradually gained over the past decade. She can't imagine where they're coming from, because she can scarcely recall the last time she enjoyed a meal. The food on her plate goes virtually untouched as she busies herself with feeding the kids, listening to her husband, and getting up to answer the phone. Her real eating is almost entirely unconscious. She'll munch on cookie dough while preparing to bake, polish off uneaten food from the children's plates while cleaning up, snack in the car while chauffeuring the kids around, and spoon ice cream directly from the carton as she flops, exhausted, in front of the television. At the end of the day, she hasn't the faintest idea what, how much or why she has eaten. Her inability to focus on eating is an expression of her overall neglect of her own needs.

• Since her mother died of cancer, Melanie has became preoccupied with her own health. She reads a lot of books on nutrition and is willing to spend more for foods that are nutritionally correct. Any food said to have disease-preventive properties gets immediately added to her diet. She plans her meals carefully to ensure that she gets her minimum daily requirement of all the nutrients she considers vital. Whether hungry or not, she eats her flax seed and oat bran muffin for breakfast, soy-based meat substitute and three veggies for lunch, and so forth. Even the ounce of dark chocolate she eats for dessert is mandated by her nutrition program: chocolate is rich in antioxidants.

• Sally was slim and unusually attractive when she married Alex five years ago. Soon after their marriage she noticed that he seemed increasingly paranoid about the many admiring glances she got from other men whenever they went out. Sometimes he flew into unfounded jealous rages. Around the same time he also got in the habit of bringing home treats for her—boxes of expensive chocolates, fresh croissants, and gourmet cheeses. Although she complained that all these goodies were going to her waistline, Alex professed to like her plumper shape. The more she ate and put on weight, the less anxious and jealous he seemed. Her overeating seemed to forge some truce between them.

- Tina works long hours at a job she finds rather boring. Eating at scheduled intervals is how she breaks up the day and gives herself something to look forward to. She spends the first two hours of the workday anticipating her midmorning yogurt break. After that snack, it's another two hours 'til lunch. The long afternoon is punctuated by a trip to the coffee bar for a latte and a later trip to the vending machines for a small pack of chips. Eating also structures her time at home. Whenever she doesn't know what else to do with herself, she moseys into the kitchen to see if the fridge has any suggestions.

Chapter 4 | Inaccurate Eating

What all these people have in common is that they are eating for reasons other than hunger. Those reasons are as individual as the people them selves. Some of them are obviously emotional: Emily's unresolved autonomy issues, Billy's homesickness, and the unconscious attempts of Alex and Katrina to solve their respective marital difficulties with food. But other reasons seem more practical than emotional: Jessica's eating for energy, Melanie's eating for health, Stan's preventative eating before he boards a flight. Some reasons are linked to personal identity and beliefs, like George's economy eating, Amy's "I'm not-a-problem-child" eating, and Erica's live-life-to-the-fullest eating. And some reasons are scarcely reasons at all. They are just unexamined habits, like Tina's use of food to fill and structure time, or Myra's mindless grazing.

For the most part, the people I've described are not bingeing or stuffing themselves to any outrageous degree. What makes them overeaters is not the *amount* that they are eating but their *reasons* for eating. They are using food to solve problems or meet needs that have nothing to do with hunger. This leads them to eat at times when their bodies don't need any food, or to go on eating after their hunger has been satisfied. In other words, they are eating *inaccurately.*

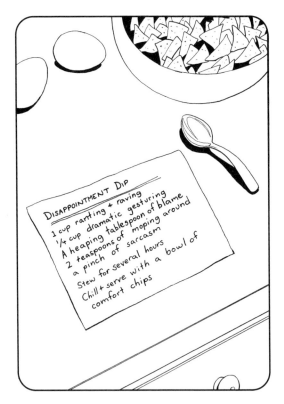

Sheila couldn't decide whether to bring the
vegetable platter or the disappointment dip.

Food is just fuel

If the only benefit we ever received from eating was to replenish spent nutrients, we could all be perfectly happy subsisting on flavorless diet shakes for the rest of our lives. Obviously most of us can't. Food nourishes the soul as well as the body. It is rich in memories and emotional associations. It comforts, pleases, and amuses us. Thin people, too, have these feelings about food.

When I insist that food is just fuel, I'm not suggesting that you should take a Spartan attitude toward it, denying all the sensory and emotional gratification it gives you. Trouble only arises when you seek this gratification in the absence of physical hunger. If you're longing for mac & cheese, mashed potatoes, or a chili dog because of the happy emotional associations you have with these foods, by all means indulge. Just wait till you're really hungry to do so. When you follow your thintuition, you can be a gourmet, a vegan, or a junk food junkie—whatever floats your boat. As long as you are physically hungry when you sit down to eat—and you stop eating as soon as your hunger stops—your whims are law.

Recognizing that many of us are driven to overeat by deep-seated emotional conflicts, some experts maintain that you will not succeed in managing your weight until you get to the root of the trouble. It is true that if you are eating to solve some problem other than hunger, that problem may clamor for attention as soon as you stop overeating. If you want to eat because you feel lonely, sad, or bored, yet realize that you're not really hungry, you will have to find some other way of addressing those emotional needs. Learning to follow your thintuition may bring buried issues to the surface and precipitate some emotional discomfort.

Still, I don't believe that your efforts to eat mindfully have to be placed on hold until you've worked through every difficulty and received a clean bill of psychological health. My own initial experience was that thintuition itself went a long way toward alleviating the issues that drove my overeating. At the root of many weight problems is a tendency to disregard one's own needs and feelings and to surrender one's autonomy. This leads to wild fluctuations between self-indulgence and self-denial—neither of which is emotionally nourishing. To follow your thintuition is to reclaim your autonomy and consistently honor your true needs. It is a way of being very good to yourself. This concentration on identifying what you truly need and want is both wise and kind, and can work wonders with whatever it is that ails you emotionally.

Being wise and kind with yourself includes dealing wisely and kindly with your lapses. When you begin to practice thintuition, you may find that you sometimes give in to strong desires for food at moments when you're not really hungry. These slip-ups are an opportunity to learn more about the needs and feelings that tempt you to overeat. If you have eaten in the absence of hunger, ask yourself why. Don't pass judgment on the reason. Simply note it. You will begin to notice patterns. Perhaps you are most likely to overeat at the end of a stressful day, or when you suffer a disappointment, or when offered food that's just too delicious to pass up. Once you identify your personal triggers, you can develop tactics for coping with them.

Let me stress one more time that when I speak of overeating, I'm not talking about the *amount* you eat, per se. Overeating is not about how many calories, carbs, or fats you consume, how frequently you eat, or what size portions you eat. It's about your *motives* for eating. To eat a carrot stick when you're not hungry is overeating. To eat a slice of carrot cake when you're legitimately hungry is not.

But how do you know when you're hungry? How do you know when your body has had enough? These questions are not as dumb as they might sound at first. We'll tackle them in the next chapter.

◆

To follow your thintuition is to reclaim your autonomy and consistently honor your true needs.

◆

Chapter 5

Satisfying Your Hunger

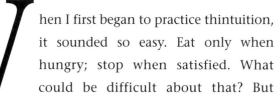hen I first began to practice thintuition, it sounded so easy. Eat only when hungry; stop when satisfied. What could be difficult about that? But on the very first day, I encountered an unexpected snag. I realized that I didn't really *know* when I was hungry, or when I'd had enough. Oddly enough, I wasn't sure what hunger felt like. All my life, I'd been saying, "I'm hungry" because that's what you say before you eat. Hunger, for me, was simply the intention to eat. I could not immediately connect with the physiological state Bob Schwartz seemed to have in mind.

I've since discovered that I'm not unusual in this. Overweight people have a lot of trouble connecting with their bodies in general, and with the sensation of hunger in particular.

When you're heavier than you want to be, you have a lot of good reasons to disengage from your body. For one thing, you probably don't really *like* your body. You are displeased with the way it looks, and you may have disagreeable sensations, such as feeling winded when you climb a few flights of stairs, or chafed by clothes that don't fit you well. The size of your body makes you feel self-conscious at times, and stands in the way of things you'd like to do.

You probably also distrust your body. You are dismayed at how quickly it puts on weight the moment you relax your vigilance. You have come to think of your body as a big problem that can only be solved by doing things you wish you didn't have to do. Hunger, in particular, is a sensation you distrust. If you're trying to stick to a diet, hunger is synonymous with temptation. It makes you want to eat at times when you're not supposed to, or to indulge in foods that you're not supposed to have. In your mind, hunger is what happens just before you break your latest resolution.

Besides dreading what hunger might make them do, a lot of overweight people are mildly anxious about the sensation of hunger in and of itself. Asked to describe it, they will use words that apply to illness or distress—words like "pang." They conceive of it as a kind of trouble the body is in, rather than as a healthy and natural occurrence. For many overweight people, hunger is so often linked to anxiety that the two feelings have become intertwined. Not only do you feel anxious when hungry, but you tend to assume you're hungry whenever you feel anxious. This is not merely due to trying to solve emotional problems with food, as we described in the previous chapter. It's a more fundamental confusion about your physical experience. Emotions cause physical sensations, and you may have learned to mislabel some of these sensations as "hunger."

True hunger is difficult to describe in words. It is a physical sensation accompanied by the desire to eat and, quite often, a specific idea of what you want to eat. Naturally thin people are never in doubt of these signals because physical hunger is the *only* reason food ever crosses their minds. If they're wanting food, they must be hungry—end of discussion. For inaccurate eaters, it's a bit trickier, because they are used to thinking about food and desiring food for reasons other than physical hunger.

To get in touch with real hunger, you also need to learn what hunger is *not*. So let's look at some of the sensations that inaccurate eaters often confuse with hunger.

Abdominal discomfort

Real hunger doesn't cause stomach pain or "pangs" until it has become quite advanced. After three days without food, your stomach might hurt, but it shouldn't hurt if you've just missed lunch. Excess acid will cause a gnawing sensation that seems to be relieved, at least temporarily, by eating. But excess stomach acid is not the same as hunger. Often it is caused by stress, and it may also be caused by chronic overeating. When you are truly hungry, the stomach merely feels empty—that is, you no longer feel in it the presence of the last meal you ate. Your belly may also make rumbling or gurgling noises.

Feeling empty

Sadness, loneliness, and boredom may all be accompanied by a physical sensation that feels like something is missing. It might feel almost like there's a gaping hole in your gut. This isn't hunger. When you perceive that the stomach is *literally* empty, you feel neutral about it on an emotional level. The emptiness is a merely a fact, not a source of distress or discontent. Many thin people actually enjoy the light feeling they have on an empty stomach.

Low energy

Food provides energy, so it's natural to assume you're hungry when your energy seems low. And sometimes you truly are. But energy drops have many possible causes, including eating *too much.* Your energy may be low because you're bored, because you're trying to suppress a strong emotion, because you've been sitting still too long, because you need some fresh air, or because you're just plain tired.

Irritability and distraction

When hunger has reached a fairly advanced stage, you may feel short-tempered, or spacey, or have difficulty concentrating. As with low energy, there are a host of other reasons why you might be feeling this way.

Thirst

The body needs fluids more often and more urgently than it needs food, and the sensation of thirst may be difficult to distinguish from hunger. Often when we are thirsty, we feel vaguely "draggy" without feeling especially dry in the mouth or throat. If you're not sure whether you feel hungry or thirsty, the easiest way to find out is to drink a glass of water. Thirst symptoms disappear immediately as soon as you have something to drink.

The best way to learn your body's genuine hunger signals is to get hungry on purpose and observe what happens. Thin people have lots of direct experience of hunger to draw on, because they don't especially mind hunger or rush to relieve it. This is usually not the case with inaccurate eaters, however. They tend to overreact to the first signs of hunger, relieving it before they've had time to fully experience what it feels like. Some inaccurate eaters *never* get truly hungry, because they are eating so often to meet needs other than hunger.

The human body can survive for many weeks without food. There's nothing dangerous about missing a meal. It won't even cause you serious discomfort. Mind you, I'm not recommending that you start skipping meals as a method of weight control. I'm simply pointing out that hunger isn't an emergency. Unless you're diabetic, letting yourself get a little hungrier than you're used to isn't going to do you any harm. Prolong your hunger just enough to learn what it feels like, how it differs from your other impulses to eat—and to get over your fear of it. Try postponing a meal for an hour or so, or skipping a habitual snack, and pay close attention to what you experience in your body.

When you get in touch with your actual hunger, you may make some surprising discoveries about it. For example, you may find that it doesn't correspond to your current meal schedule, or that your hunger levels fluctuate from day to day. I must admit that I'm still surprised sometimes when

I come home from a ten-mile run and don't feel especially hungry. Having burned up all that energy, why doesn't my body need more? And why do I sometimes find myself unusually hungry the next day, when I'm still recovering from my workout and not exerting myself much? There's probably a scientific explanation, but I don't know what it is. All I know is that when I eat in accordance with my *actual* hunger—as opposed to my *idea* of how hungry I should or shouldn't be— I'm able to maintain my ideal weight without a struggle.

Good to be full?

A famously skinny actress had to gain thirty pounds for a role. When asked in an interview how she would go about losing the excess weight after the film, she replied, "I'll just go back to doing what I like to do. I like to stop eating when I've had enough."

To the inaccurate eater, that statement is all but unintelligible. She *likes* to stop? Stopping feels *good*? If eating is a pleasure, where is the pleasure in stopping?

Most naturally thin people enjoy their food every bit as much as overweight people do. In fact, many enjoy it more, because they eat whatever they really want, without inhibition or self-reproach. The difference is that they also enjoy being finished. They like the feeling they get when they have eaten exactly enough to satisfy their hunger, and not a bite more. They strongly dislike the way they feel when they have eaten more than enough.

Inaccurate eaters, on the other hand, tend to feel that they haven't finished eating if they still "have room." They have learned to tolerate the sensation of fullness, or even to enjoy it. The tag line of a recent commercial—"It's good to be full"—is the overeater's motto. The very word "full" has positive connotations for them. It may be subconsciously connected with other feelings or conditions such as completion, abundance, success, strength, generosity, stability, or tranquility. Some overweight people can't feel connected with their body at all unless they are full. When they don't have a sensation of heaviness in the belly, they feel as if they're not quite "all there." What thin people often especially dislike about fullness—feeling heavy, dull, and groggy—may be perceived as a benefit by someone who is driven to overeat by anxiety or stress. Being full has a sedative effect.

Diets appeal to this desire to feel full when they promise that you can eat unlimited quantities of certain foods. Confusing satisfaction with fullness also leads some people to believe they need gastric bypass surgery. Convinced that to satisfy one's hunger means eating until there's no more room, they discard part of the stomach so that there will be less room available. Minuscule amounts of food will then produce the desired feeling of fullness. This drastic and potentially dangerous "solution" is based on an equally drastic misunderstanding of the real problem. If your weight problem is severe enough to qualify you for such surgery, the issue you need to come to grips with is your compulsion to feel full. Healthy people dislike that feeling, and you can retrain yourself to dislike it, too.

Satisfaction is different from fullness. When your body has gotten as much food as it needs for the present, it stops sending hunger signals. This usually occurs before the stomach is completely full, so it doesn't matter how big your stomach is, or how much room you have left. Eating has accomplished its purpose: you're no longer hungry. That means you're finished, regardless of how much more food you could cram in if you really tried.

The moment of satisfaction is subtle. It is the absence of the strong feeling that initially drove you to eat, rather than an equally strong *new* feeling like fullness. Most overeaters fail to perceive the moment of satisfaction because they are busy pursuing fullness. By the time you notice that your belly feels heavy or your belt is getting tight, you are well *beyond* the satisfaction point.

Getting satisfaction

One of the great ironies of being overweight is that inaccurate eaters think about food quite often when they're not really hungry, yet have tremendous difficulty focusing on food while they're actually eating it. You could even say that the problem of overweight people is that they don't enjoy eating *enough*. That's why they don't perceive the moment of satisfaction—their attention is elsewhere when it occurs.

To be unable to focus on the act of eating is another symptom of overall disconnection from the body. It may have something to do with shame. A lot of overweight people feel they need to conceal what they're really eating, or how much they're really eating. They tend to eat relatively little when around other people, then indulge in what they *really* want to eat when alone. Yet these moments of indulgence are rarely savored. You may eat standing by the fridge, or while engaged in something else like driving, watching television, reading, or working at your desk. Distracting yourself from the act of eating keeps you from fully registering what you are doing and feeling guilty about it. Alas, distracting yourself also prevents you from fully *enjoying* your food. The pleasure you might be getting from it is largely wasted because your have detached from your physical senses. You may be eating too much because the enjoyment you expect to get from food keeps eluding you.

Strange as it might sound, to succeed with thintuition, you will need to learn to take more pleasure in eating. You may end up eating smaller quantities, but you won't feel deprived because you will be getting so much more enjoyment than you used to. Until you learn to relish the act of eating, wholeheartedly and single-mindedly, you will continue to have difficulty identifying the exact moment to stop.

Until now, I've refrained from offering direct advice. My whole point has been that you need to stop listening to advice and start listening to your own instincts. But after a lifetime of learning to worry, obsess, and berate yourself about food, you might need a little coaching in how to really savor the experience of eating. So I'm going to make some recommendations. These are not rules, and you might not practice them all the time or for the rest of your life. They're just some specific behavior changes that have helped me and others tune in to the experience of satisfaction and identify the moment to quit.

- Treat every morsel of food you consume as an official meal. Even if it's just a cookie or an apple, sit down at a table and put it on a plate. Approach it with a sense of ceremony.

- Give eating your undivided attention. If you're eating alone, don't watch television or read. Just be with yourself. Dining with others is a bit trickier, because obviously you can't completely ignore them. But keep bringing your attention back to your food whenever there's a lull in the conversation, or let your companions do most of the talking.

- Go slowly. Put your fork down between bites. Savor the flavor, the aroma, the act of chewing. Notice how your whole body feels, not just your mouth. Notice how pleasurably it responds when the food you have chosen is exactly what it was wanting.

- Eat first what appeals to you most. Your policy from now on is "pleasure before duty." Don't save the best for last, because you may run out of hunger before you get to it and then be tempted to overeat. If your favorite part of fried chicken is the skin, go for it. If you want to pick all the cheese off your pizza and leave the crust behind, you're entitled. Don't put anything into your mouth that doesn't taste wonderful. Eat like a child whose parents are away. You don't have to finish your peas to earn your dessert.

Chapter 5 | **Satisfying Your Hunger**

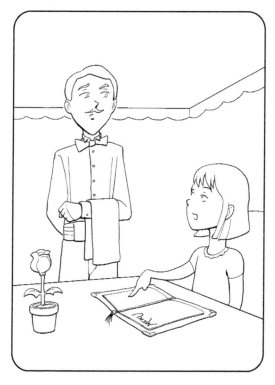

"I'll have the crème brûlée."

- Don't sweat portion size. How much food a restaurant puts on your plate or what a food package defines as a single serving is completely irrelevant to how much you need to eat. If you've taken or been served too much, you don't have to finish it. If you've taken too little, you can always have seconds. You are *never* obliged to clean your plate. Instead of defining food you leave uneaten as "wasted," consider it evidence of your newfound accuracy. (If you feel guilty about throwing away food when people in the world are starving, donate to famine relief. Overeating isn't going to help those unfortunate people in Ethiopia.)

- How hungry you feel at the start of a meal is not always a reliable guide to how much you will need to eat. You never know that for certain until you're actually eating. You might feel like you could eat a horse and sit down to one, only to find that your hunger has abated much faster than you expected. Or your hunger might be fairly modest, so you figure you are eating accurately when you order just an appetizer. But modest as it seems, the appetizer might actually be too much. It's *eating* accurately, not *ordering* accurately, that will make you slim. Order or cook as much as you feel you want, but commit yourself only on a bite-by-bite basis.

• If you sometimes overeat to flatter the cook, pay tribute with your pleasure instead. Make a big deal of savoring the food. Praise it extravagantly instead of eating it extravagantly.

• Notice how taste and your other sensory experiences change over the course of the meal. As the saying goes, "Hunger is the best sauce"—meaning that the first few bites you take are often the most delicious. When the flavors come to seem less intense, or a tad repetitive, that's a sign that your hunger has diminished.

• Notice how your energy level changes. The act of digestion itself requires energy—which is why you feel sluggish or sleepy after eating too much. When you first start to eat, it may be a struggle to make yourself go slowly, for your whole body feels energetic and eager. But once the edge is off your hunger, your energy level declines slightly. This subtle feeling of slowing down usually begins before you are full, and is a good indication that you've eaten enough.

- Keep asking yourself, "Do I feel hungry?" At the beginning of the meal, it will seem like a silly question. It will get harder to answer as your hunger diminishes and its signals become more subtle. At the point when you can no longer detect the feeling of hunger, consider yourself a bite or two away from complete satisfaction. Savor those last two bites, then stop.

- You might be tempted to go on eating past the point of satisfaction because you're still really enjoying the food. You'll enjoy it even more if you save it for when you get hungry again. This is why Tupperware, doggie bags, and microwave ovens were invented.

- You might be anxious that if you don't feel full, you haven't really eaten enough, and will soon be hungry again. Eat only to satisfy the hunger you feel right now, not to forestall future hunger. Be happy that you're going to get hungry again! Feeling hunger more keenly than you're used to is a sign that your metabolism is starting to work better. There is no reason to dread your hunger, for you have promised yourself to enjoy the food you want every time your body asks for it. Letting yourself get good and hungry first will enhance your pleasure.

The Hunger Guide

Naturally thin people are precise about hunger and fullness. Where an overweight person generally just says, "I'm hungry, time to eat," a naturally thin person makes subtle distinctions like, "I'm a little bit hungry, but not ready to drop what I'm doing yet." Or, "I'm starting to get hungry, but this airplane food doesn't appeal to me. I think I'll wait and have something after we land." Or, "I can't finish a whole dessert but I want just a bite of something really rich and gooey." It is this level of precision about how they're really feeling that enables thin people to fully satisfy their hunger every single time without overeating.

The difference between your current weight and your ideal weight often amounts to no more than a few bites too many at every meal, or a modest amount of between-meal nibbling when you're not hungry. Recognizing this, some weight control experts will recommend minor but permanent "lifestyle" changes, such as giving up your afternoon cookie or your bedtime snack. Trouble is, you might actually be hungry for that cookie some afternoons. The source of your unwanted girth might not be the "empty calories" in the cookie at all. It might be the salad you oblige yourself to eat with every dinner because you think you're supposed to, or the nutritious breakfast you force down when you're not hungry. It might be the leftovers of a meal you wanted very much yesterday and now don't especially care for, or the popcorn you were hungry for when you entered the theater then went on mindlessly eating once you got caught up in the movie. The only way to know for sure is to pay close attention to your hunger levels throughout the day, each and every day.

While working to develop my thintuition, I found it helpful to assign a numerical rating to my hunger level before, during, and after each meal. By doing so, I learned to make the subtle distinctions that thin people make automatically. Between meals, the numbers helped me differentiate between early "some food would be nice" hunger and fully developed "gotta eat *now*" hunger. Continuing to rate my hunger throughout a meal taught me to identify the exact moment when I was satisfied, when any more than one more bite would put me into the fullness range. I've turned my rating system into a handy chart, called the Hunger Guide, which is illustrated on the following page. On the thintuition website (www.thintuition.com), you can print a full-color version for free, or purchase other versions of it in various formats—a credit card size to slip into your wallet, a tent card to display on your dining table, or a moveable wheel that reminds you of the physical signs that accompany each level of hunger and satisfaction.

hunger guide

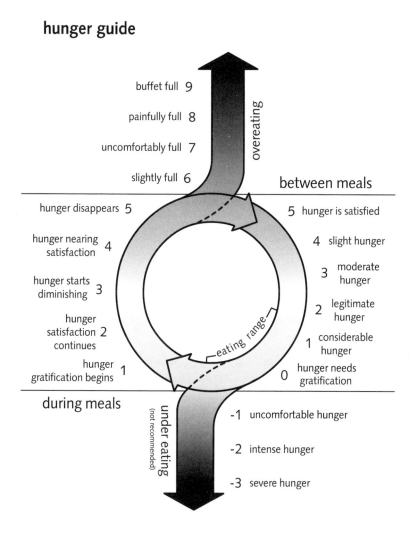

buffet full 9

painfully full 8

uncomfortably full 7

slightly full 6

overeating

between meals

hunger disappears 5

5 hunger is satisfied

hunger nearing satisfaction 4

4 slight hunger

hunger starts diminishing 3

3 moderate hunger

hunger satisfaction 2 continues

2 legitimate hunger

hunger gratification begins 1

1 considerable hunger

eating range

0 hunger needs gratification

during meals

under eating (not recommended)

-1 uncomfortable hunger

-2 intense hunger

-3 severe hunger

While trying to make a permanent behavior change, it is helpful to track your progress. When you keep a record, you are less likely to eat mindlessly or to lie to yourself about your eating habits. From the perspective of thintuition, there are no wrong food choices, so counting calories, fat grams, or portion sizes is counterproductive. The Hunger Guide gives you a more meaningful set of numbers to jot in your diary. You can record your hunger levels at the start and finish of each meal. When you find that you've eaten your way into the fullness range, you can jot down the reason, look for patterns in these reasons, and address the underlying problem.

Track your hunger levels throughout the day, but *don't* keep track of what or how much you are eating. Remember that overeating is about *why* you are eating, not what you are eating or how much. In eating mindfully, your goal is not necessarily to eat less. It's to eat *exactly* what your hunger requires. If you are eating only when really hungry and stopping as soon as your hunger ceases, you are eating the right amount for your body. Rating your hunger levels will help keep the focus where it belongs—on your physical experience, not your food.

Occasionally you may realize you're on the verge of fullness and choose to go on eating anyhow. Even thin people do so once in a great while. In the beginning, you may also overeat by accident, because you haven't yet learned to distinguish satisfaction from fullness, or because you're eating too fast, or because your attention wanders at some point during a meal. These lapses are a great opportunity to focus on how fullness really feels. Once you have some experiences of being satisfied without being full, you can compare and contrast. Notice what's unpleasant about being full— the bloatedness, the dullness and sluggishness, the possible indigestion, the feeling that what you ate two hours ago is still lingering in your stomach. Compare this with how you feel when you've left the table after eating exactly enough and no more. Eventually you'll be able to understand how that skinny actress could say, "I like to stop when I've had enough."

◆

In eating mindfully,
your goal
is not necessarily
to eat less.
It's to eat *exactly* what
your hunger requires.

◆

Chapter 6
The Art and Skill of thintuition

Maybe what we are really seeking when we cram in all the food our stomachs will hold is not fullness, but *wholeness*. I know that in my years of dieting, I never felt whole—not even in the triumphant moments of reaching my goal weight. I had this sense that, regardless of what I weighed, I never seemed to come together as my complete and authentic self. My beliefs, intentions, desires, and actions were all skidding off in umpteen different and contradictory directions. I felt I wasn't meeting my full potential in *any* aspect of my life. My fluctuating weight mirrored my inner restlessness and uncertainty.

Dieting does that to people. It causes fragmentation. To the extent that you accept the propaganda about food and weight circulating in the culture at large, you find yourself with a vast assortment of ideas and beliefs. Some of these beliefs are mutually exclusive and many of them are flatly contradicted by your own experience. But that doesn't stop you from entertaining them. The beliefs give rise to all sorts of resolutions, many of which are incompatible with your desires, your natural instincts, and the way your body actually functions. Because the resolutions don't make a lot of sense to begin with, they can't be kept for long and they lead to contradictory behaviors. You alternately starve yourself and binge. The resulting failures lead to a whole new round of conflicting beliefs. ("I'm undisciplined and self-indulgent." "I can't help being overweight. It's genetic.")

The hallmark of whole people—people of power and integrity—is that their beliefs align with their conscious intentions, and their intentions align with their actions. What they believe, they resolve, and what they resolve, they do. Conviction, desire, and behavior all add up to one seamless whole, moving in a single, consistent direction. I recovered this wholeness when I resolved never to diet again and began to practice thintuition. To act on my commitments was never a struggle, because these commitments were based on reality and fully compatible with both my conscious desires and my unconscious instincts. The stable and trim weight that resulted mirrored both the consistency and the newfound simplicity of my inner life. As I cleared out the clutter of diet propaganda that had expanded to fill every available convolution of my brain, the fat went away with it.

Chapter 6 | The Art and Skill of thintuition

You may be wondering whether this is the chapter where I'm finally going to tell you how much weight you can expect to lose, and how fast. It isn't. I can't tell you, because I honestly don't know. What I do know is that any "expert" who tells you what weight you will attain and how fast you'll get there is just spitting into the wind. Your body is the sole expert on what it wants to weigh and how quickly or slowly it wants to move toward getting there. Your body's primary agenda is to be healthy. It will seek the weight that is good for it at a pace that is good for it.

I was frankly surprised by how many pounds I lost, how fast they came off, and how firmly I stabilized at my ideal weight. Having never before achieved my ideal, I was prepared to settle for less. I was fully committed to practicing thintuition for the rest of my days even if the results were modest, because I believed it was right. I was committed to respecting and trusting my body's natural wisdom—whatever the resulting weight—because I had resolved once and for all to respect and trust *myself*. I believed that this was how to treat myself right.

And I think that's really the point. If you go into this because you believe—or at least hope—you will get someone else's best-case-scenario result, your commitment to it is conditional. As long as the pounds are melting away at the hoped-for rate, you'll be a thintuition fanatic. But if the results come too slowly, or you hit a plateau, you mentally reserve the right to bail on thintuition and resort to cabbage soup, compulsive workouts, or gastric bypass surgery. That's the same-old same-old diet mentality. When you focus entirely on results, part of you is preparing to repudiate your latest diet plan before you've even started. From the outset of every weight loss program, you're envisioning the day you will go off it.

That secret intention to bail out eventually is your common sense talking. You *should* quit when what you've undertaken isn't good for you in the first place. Yet the lack of full and permanent commitment is what ultimately dooms your weight loss attempts. You will not be able to maintain a stable and healthy weight until you discover the resolutions that are truly right for you—commitments that express what you desire, what you believe to be true, and what you are actually capable of doing. Treating yourself right is the only plan your body and your psyche will stand for on a permanent basis.

Reclaiming your birthright

The point of thintuition is not how thin you might become in the future. Thintuition is about reconnecting with who you really are, about awakening the healthy instincts you *already* have.

Chapter 6 | The Art and Skill of thintuition

Everybody is born with thintuition. Even if you weighed twelve pounds at birth, you had it. You cried to be fed whenever you were hungry, and you lost all interest in feeding the moment your hunger was satisfied. You eagerly ate whatever you desired, and spat out anything you didn't need or want. If you've ever tried feeding an infant or toddler who doesn't feel like eating, you'll know what I'm talking about.

Until very recently in human history, obesity was rare. Almost everyone was of normal weight, provided there was enough food around. If they had any weight-related health concern at all, it was worry about being too skinny. Now, it is true that the human body might change *gradually* due to evolution, but gradually is the operative word. A marked evolutionary change doesn't happen in a generation, or a century. You have the same kind of body people used to have back when nobody was worried about getting fat.

Your weight problem is the result of the culture you're living in, not the biology you were born with. The culture has taught you to base your eating on ideas rather than on natural inclinations, and a lot of those ideas are just plain silly. The scientific assumptions and procedures on which they're based are of very recent invention. If our survival depended on all this science, humanity would long ago have gone the way of the dinosaur.

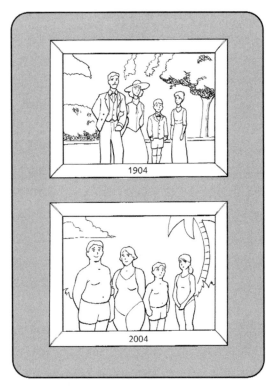

The Smith family's genetics mysteriously
changed over time.

Thintuition is not about what you are trying to become. It's about realizing who and what you already are. You are a person who was born knowing what you need, a person whose natural instincts still gravitate toward what will make your body healthy. Regardless of how you may appear on the outside, deep down you are naturally thin. You don't need to change your basic nature. You just need to stop interfering with nature by confusing hunger and its satisfaction with all manner of irrelevant ideas and agendas.

You've probably long been in the habit of telling yourself the opposite. You say to yourself, "I'm too fat," or "I can't seem to lose weight no matter how hard I try," or "If I eat those fries, they're going to go straight to my thighs." Self-talk of any kind tends to be self-fulfilling, so if you keep making negative assertions, negative results are hardly surprising. The unsatisfactory appearance of your body reflects the unsatisfactory nature of your thoughts. Positive assertions work just as efficiently to bring positive results—the more so if these positive assertions happen to be true.

Thintuition is not about what you are trying to become. It's about realizing who and what you already are.

This book has had a lot to say about the kind of assertions you need to abandon. Now I'm going to offer you six simple thoughts with which to replace them, six assertions that express the truth about the nature you were born with. All six describe this truth in *behavioral* terms. When you think the truth, speak the truth, and act on the truth, your entire being is properly aligned. You are whole. You make sense. Your outward appearance will come to reflect the beliefs that you put into practice, because that's what bodies do. It's what your body has been doing all along.

The Six Practices of People Who Follow Their thintuition

 ### 1 distinguish between appetite and hunger.

Hunger is the physical need for food. Appetite is the desire for the sensory pleasure and emotional gratification we get from food. When hunger and appetite coincide, it's time to eat. But as you well know, it is possible to experience appetite when you're not actually hungry. Your body doesn't need food right now, but you want some anyhow.

As a person who follows your thintuition, you can tell the difference. You say to yourself, "That bacon smells fantastic. But I'm not really hungry right now." Or, "It's noon and I need a break. But I don't feel hungry for lunch." Or, "I'm feeling emotionally empty and I seem to need something. But I'm not physically hungry." You are not confused by irrelevant impulses to eat, because you are able to distinguish appetite from genuine hunger.

I eat to satisfy physical hunger.

As a person who follows your thintuition, you act on your ability to recognize when you are truly hungry. You trust your body's hunger signals and treat them with respect. If you are hungry, you eat. You don't care whether it's an official mealtime or not. Your body needs food, so you give it some. You take care of yourself that way. When you'd like some food, but don't feel truly hungry, you wait. You don't burden your body with food it can't use out of needs or desires that have nothing to do with physical hunger.

I eat the foods I desire.

As a person who follows your thintuition, you eat what you really want—and only what you really want—every single time you get hungry. You regard hunger as a precious resource, too valuable to waste on foods you don't care for.

You eat what you like best for two very good reasons. First, you know that constantly depriving yourself exaggerates your desire for certain foods, setting you up for a binge. Desires that are constantly denied gain power, leading eventually to rebellion and overindulgence. You don't put yourself in that situation, because you don't pass judgment on your desires. When you feel hungry, you don't go looking for reasons to deny yourself what you really want.

Secondly, and more importantly, you trust your body to know best what it needs. If it's low on protein, it will alert you by making you hungry for a protein food. If it requires a certain vitamin, foods rich in that vitamin will appeal to you. You know that if you get in the habit of ignoring or denying your desire for foods you consider to be frivolous, you won't hear your body when it tries to tell you it needs spinach. You don't deliberate a lot about nutrition. You just trust that your body's natural desire for a variety of foods will lead you reliably to the nutrients you need.

I savor each and every bite.

Because you embrace the experience of hunger and the food preferences that arise from it, you thoroughly enjoy satisfying your hunger. When the time comes to provide your body with what it needs, nothing is more important. You give the matter your full attention. You don't let yourself be distracted by competing activities, or avert your attention out of shame. You focus single-mindedly on satisfying your hunger and enjoying every step of the process.

Because you savor every bite of your food, you rarely overeat by accident. You experience the way each bite is moving you away from hunger and toward satisfaction. You can pinpoint the exact moment when your body has had enough.

Truly relishing your food enables you to be satisfied with less. Instead of bolting down a pint of ice cream, your attention wandering, your enjoyment dulled by self-reproach, you fully experience the sweetness, the creaminess, the melting in your mouth. From a half-cup of ice cream you derive more gratification than overeaters get from polishing off the entire carton.

1 regard food as fuel.

Pleasure is a byproduct of eating, and an important one. But there's a big difference between a byproduct and a *purpose*. The only purpose of eating is to replenish the nutrients and energy your body uses up.

As a person who follows your thintuition, you understand that food is just fuel. Any other meanings food has acquired for you are incidental. These meanings may enhance your pleasure in consuming what your body needs. But you recognize that they would become harmful if they led you to consume food it doesn't need.

Because you get that food is just fuel, you are struck by the weirdness of the contrary messages that constantly bombard you via the media. You notice how advertisers keep trying to entice you to equate foods with irrelevant emotions and conditions—fun, togetherness, self-reward, prosperity, relaxation, economy, strength, health, or athletic prowess. You see how medical science, as reported by the media, assails you with equally irrelevant hopes and fears, promising that certain foods will enhance your longevity, lower your cholesterol, or improve your memory, while warning that other foods will give you everything from zits to cancer. You notice, too, how sometimes your own mind proposes food as a solution to problems that have nothing to do with hunger. But you're not taken in. You are clear that hunger is the only problem food has ever solved for you.

 # I stop eating when my hunger disappears.

As a person who follows your thintuition, you eat exactly as much food as you need to satisfy your hunger, and not a bite more. Because you are paying close attention to the process of eating, you notice how your hunger diminishes a little with each mouthful. You notice when your body has stopped sending hunger signals, and you are aware that this moment occurs before it starts sending fullness signals. You are aware that you are satisfied well before your belt starts feeling tight, well before you feel heavy, dull, or sleepy from having overeaten.

Most importantly, when you notice that you are no longer feeling hungry, you stop eating. You have learned to dislike the sensation of being full as much as you like the pleasure of eating. Knowing that you're not going to like the way you feel afterward, you resist the temptation to keep eating just because it tastes good. While in the long run you know that overeating will make you fat, your more immediate motivation is simply not to feel stuffed. You stop eating because you don't want to feel that way.

Your outward appearance will come to reflect the beliefs that you put into practice, because that's what bodies do.

Frequently asked questions

A FAQ is usually just what it sounds like—a list of questions that have been asked repeatedly, with corresponding answers. I could probably list a good hundred or so questions that have been put to me by private clients and attendees at my thintuition seminars. But the answer to nearly all of them is the same. It is (drum roll, please):

"Why are you asking me?"

For example, there's a whole category of questions concerning the relative merits of various foods. "Is it really okay to eat _____ ?" (Fill in the blank with whatever delicious food you imagine you need permission to enjoy.) How would I know whether it's okay for you to eat donuts or nachos or deep-fried pork rinds? You're the only one who knows whether you're hungry. You're the only one who knows what you're hungry *for*. What you choose to put in your stomach is no business of mine.

Chapter 6 | The Art and Skill of thintuition

Another category of questions concerns frequency of eating. "How long should I go without eating?" "Is it okay to eat six times a day?" Again, how would I know? You're the only one who knows how often you get hungry, or how long you can stay hungry and still function well.

Then there are questions about exercise. "Can I eat more if I work out?" Beats me. Are you hungrier after a workout? "Do I need to exercise at all?" Well, *do* you? If your body wants exercise, it will tell you. It won't tell me.

Having come to the end of this book, you have by now heard everything I have to tell you about thintuition as a method of managing weight. The essence of it is to listen to your own body and follow its guidance. Your body will tell you everything you need to know about how to keep it healthy, happy, and attractive. Looking for answers from anyone else—including myself—disempowers you and keeps you stuck.

Helping others to manage their weight is my life's mission. In the course of pursuing it, I've had to give a lot of thought to the question of what "help" consists of. The last thing this world needs is one more blowhard posing as a weight loss expert. The problem for most overweight Americans is too *much* information, not too little of it.

What most people seem to need, as they work on developing their thintuition, is support in *un*learning, in forgetting or ignoring all the misleading ideas they've already absorbed until now. Many also find they need social support. The two needs are linked. The culture relentlessly bombards us with unhelpful ideas about food, weight, and health, and many of these ideas carry a powerful emotional charge. No sooner do you resolve to eat what you really want than you switch on the television and hear that what you really want to eat will make you fat or sick. You can't help but feel anxious, mistrustful of your own desires. Or, just when you've resolved to give up dieting for good, you hear of some new diet that's producing spectacular results, based on some new scientific theory that sounds really persuasive. Your hopes stirred, you consider for the umpteenth time that maybe dieting does work, maybe you've just never been on the *right* diet. How can your hard-won common sense compete with all this relentless propaganda, especially when everyone around you seems to believe it? To connect with people who think like you do can be a big help in resisting the insanity of the larger culture.

You have learned by now that eating for any reason other than physical hunger is overeating, but some of those reasons can feel very compelling when you try to give them up. If you've been eating out of loneliness, grief, boredom, or stress, what are you going to do instead? How are you going to handle the intense emotions that may arise when you

Chapter 6 | The Art and Skill of thintuition

stop using food as a tranquilizer? When you take control of your eating, these other troubled areas of your life may start clamoring for your attention. For this stuff, too, it helps to have social support.

Finally, it helps to share your progress and setbacks with others who are pursuing the same goal. Weighing in, commiserating, and celebrating success were aspects of formal programs like Weight Watchers that I actually enjoyed. I figured it would be great to have a place to get all that without having to subject myself to the accompanying diet mythology.

So I set one up. On the thintuition website (www.thintuition.com) you'll find a whole community of like-minded people with whom you can share via chat rooms and bulletin boards. If the main thing you want is company, just sign on and hang out. If you want a more formal program to follow, you'll find interactive lessons on the six practices, various exercises to try, a place to journal, and a personal progress chart. You can read my occasional diatribes against the diet industry, and post diatribes of your own. But the most important aspect of the site is the opportunity to connect with others who will confirm and reinforce your own natural instincts and common sense. I hope you'll join us there, and give me the pleasure of hearing your thintuition success story.

A note from Rob Stevens

I want to thank you for being open to new information, for having the courage to change your life, and for taking the first step in recovering the thintuition that you always had inside you.

Everyone possesses thintuition. It's a natural body sense—as natural as knowing whether you are hot or cold, energized or tired. But many of us have lost our connection with our natural thintuition through perpetual dieting and from listening to the overpowering megaphone of the diet industry. However, your thintuition is there—quietly waiting to be awakened.

Once reconnected with your thintuition, you will discover how natural it is and how much sense it makes. As long as you continue to follow your thintuition, you will eventually reach and maintain your natural body weight.

My best to you,

Rob Stevens

Acknowledgements

To my loving parents, Alice and Tom: Alice, you have always been my biggest fan, my main support and the foundation of my weight loss journey to freedom. I love you and thank you. And to my amazing father, Tom. You had the courage and commitment to let go of a lifetime of fears that kept you overweight and concerned for your health and well-being. I dedicate this book to you. Congratulations on your new body and life by thintuition. I told you, Dad, trust me. This stuff really works.

I want to express my gratitude to the following brilliant and talented people, who have tirelessly gone above and beyond what I've asked of them: Steve Shefler, Catherine MacCoun, Maura Junius, Julaine E. Flick, Amy Walsh, Andy Crestodina, Barrett Lombardo, Frank J. Voznak, Dirk I. Tiede, Jeff Conta, Jeffrey Dillon, and Mark Nieds.

To the many others who have supported me in my efforts to bring the thintuition philosophy to life, thank you!

Products

At **thintuition.com** you will find an online store.
Here are some of the products you will find there:

The Overfed Head: audiobook version
Listen to this book on any CD player.

The Overfed Head: e-book
An electronic version to read on your computer.

Hunger Guide slide wheel
A durable plastic slide wheel that helps you get in touch with various levels
of hunger to guide your eating.

The thintuition e-learning weight loss program
A complete online weight loss course including a wide variety of support
features. This program can be customized to fit the needs of large groups
and corporations as well.

All products are available at special discounts when purchased in bulk
quantities for health and wellness facilities, corporations, schools, groups,
and other business use. For details contact: **info@thintuition.com**

Sources

Pages 25, 26, 27, 28, 30, 33, 34, 41 & 89: Bob Schwartz. *Diets Don't Work*.
Houston, TX: Breakthru Publishing, 1996.

Pages 50, 51, 55 & 56: Ancel B. Keys, Joseph Brozek, and Austin Henschel.
The Biology of Human Starvation. Minneapolis, MN:
University of Minnesota Press, 1950.

Page 51: Study with zero, one, or two milkshakes and ice cream
(dieters and non-dieters). C. Peter Herman & Mack, Deborah Mack (1975).
Restrained and unrestrained eating. *Journal of Personality, 43,* 647–660.

Page 74: From a January 13, 2004 article posted on www.bankrate.com
by Ellen Goodstein.

Page 86: From *USA Today Snapshots* posted on Yahoo.com. February 9, 2004.
Which diet is the most popular way to lose weight? Porter Novelli, Anne R.
Carey and Gia Kereselidze.